Praise for *Jack's Story*

"I would like to give my condolences to your family as no family should have to go through what your family endured. Taking the pain from your son's story and turning it into a moving and beautifully honest book takes a lot of courage. I appreciate the bravery it took to write this book about what it is really like inside a life with glioblastoma multiforme." **Senator John McCain**

"Thank you for sharing Jack's story. I'm deeply sorry to hear about your son's journey with cancer. As you know glioblastoma cancer has touched my life and those that I love dearly. I can only imagine how difficult this process is for you and your family. It sounds like Jack was surrounded with support and indeed possessed courage at its best. I know that the grieving process never quite ends, but in due time, the thought of your son will bring a smile to your lips sooner than a tear to your eye. Our sons gave us so much more than they knew, so much for us to cherish. Our memories of them will always be with us. Please know that Jill and I will keep you in our thoughts and prayers. We're in this with you. God Bless you." **Joseph R. Biden. Jr. (Democrat front runner for US President in 2020 against Donald Trump and ex Vice President to Barrack Obama)**

"*Jack's story* is a beautiful, powerful story. The book tells of a family's love for their son and the importance both of research and of celebrating each life while we have our loved ones with us." **Greg Hunt, Federal Minister for Health, Australia**

"It is so emotional and powerful. I can't even begin to imagine what this is like, but your book gives us all a little insight. I know there is little or nothing I can do or say to help you with this grief, but we send you our love, and know that Jack will not be forgotten." **Professor Mardi Dungey, who died after a short illness in January 2019. Mardi was prepared to move mountains to get Jack back to University.**

"*Jack's Story* is gripping and confronting. Well done for having the courage to write it and get it out there in the public space. I'm sure many other families and health professionals will benefit from reading this book. It was a real tribute to Jack and also demonstrated you didn't leave a stone unturned in trying to find a solution to this aggressive cancer." **Dr Nick Cooling**

"I read *Jack's Story* in one night …couldn't put it down … and despite knowing how it all ended, I was willing there to be a twist and turn on each page that would see a miracle happen. What a truly incredible story of hope, love, courage and ultimate tragedy." **Katie Murray**

"We read your book today up until 1am as we couldn't put it down. We feel we have ridden the emotional roller coaster with you, albeit removed from our reality. It moved us both to tears throughout and we have such admiration for your courage and dogged determination to explore and uncover every possible option. Thanks for sharing and I hope in doing so paves the way for advancements in science to address this terrible disease." **Alex Rooke**

"I'm so sorry that despite all the expert advice and treatment he received that no more could be done to save him. It is stories like these, and patients like Jack, that drive us to continue our work and research and clinical trials to try to find new and better treatments to counter this awful disease. Let's hope we can make some more break throughs in memory of all the children and young adults like Jack." **Dr David Ziegler**

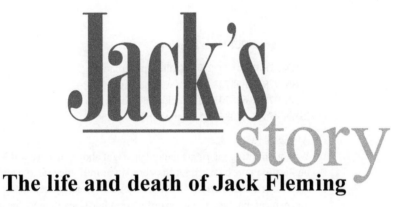

Jack's story

The life and death of Jack Fleming

His battle with a glioblastoma multiforme brain tumour

as told by his father **Ken Fleming**

Copyright © 2019 Ken Fleming

ISBN 978-0-6487032-0-4 (colour paperback)
ISBN 978-0-6487032-1-1 (b/w paperback)
ISBN 978-0-6487032-2-8 (colour hardback)
ISBN 978-0-6483457-5-6 (ebook)

Published by
K&D Publishing, Hobart, Tasmania
www.jacksstory.com.au

 A catalogue record for this
book is available from the
National Library of Australia

Design and layout by Kent Whitmore

Printed by Ingram Spark

foreword

THIS IS THE STORY OF A VERY BRAVE YOUNG MAN that I had the pleasure of sharing 21 years with because that is all that he had to share, 21 years.

I was with him when he took his first breath and I was with him when he took his last. One was a moment of exquisite pleasure and the other was a moment of unimaginable pain.

He gave life, and particularly the last two years struggling with terminal brain cancer, his best shot. He never stopped smiling; never gave up; never said no more.

He was diagnosed with glioblastoma multiforme (GBM) brain cancer on a cold, wet and wintry 8 July 2016.

He was given 12 months to live. We got 22 months. Christmas 2016 I thought would be his last Christmas and he would never see 21. However, we made it to Christmas 2017 and on 25 November, 2017, we celebrated his 21st birthday.

In December 2017, we found out that none of the treatments to date were working and he was unlikely to live much longer as the tumour was now extensive and he could "drop dead at any time".

We tried a few more things but on 28 March, 2018, we were told it was all over.

Jack died at 1.45 pm on 15 April, 2018.

I loved him from the moment Dianne conceived and I miss him every minute, of every day. As I write this it is just over one month since he died and the pain is as real and as raw now as it was on that day.

This is Jack's story. I promised him I would write the book and I also promised him I would save his life. I intend to keep one of those promises.

JACK EVAN FLEMING
25 November 1996 – 15 April 2018
RIP

Ken (Dad)

contents

introduction

THIS BOOK IS ABOUT JACK, HIS FAMILY, HIS DIAGNOSIS, struggle and death. The synopsis of the book is about his life and particularly the last 22 months. It is a love story and a tragedy and tells about an ordinary family who waged an extraordinary battle against a disease that takes no prisoners, has no foundation and no cure. Shit happens. We never stood a chance but there were times we believed we were winning. It is a story of hope and promise, as well as loss and despair, and finally, tragedy.

But we are not the only family that has suffered loss at the hands of this nefarious disease and we won't be the last. So, I have asked myself, how do I make something good come out of Jack's tragic death? How do I fill the vacuum that consumes my dear wife, my family and me? I promised Jack I would save his life and I didn't. But I also told him I would write a book and tell his story and maybe, just maybe, it will help other families in some small way.

And maybe, if the book were to be successful, I could use some of the money to find a cure for brain cancer ... Jack liked that idea and I remember the warmth of his smile.

He didn't like being the centre of attention and the old Jack would have resisted vehemently any suggestion that he would be the subject of a book. But as the disease progressed we both fooled each other that we would find a way out of this maze and it would make great copy and we would become enormously wealthy and he wouldn't have to worry about working again. And that was an increasing frustration for him as his natural brilliance was slowly suffocated by the disease, the drugs, the surgeries and the radiation. "I am now the dumbest person in the family" he would lament.

He was not the dumbest and probably was the smartest, but as the tumour crushed his brain his smarts were crushed too. Get rid of the tumour and a lot of that brain function would come back but not all of it. There were bits missing because of surgery and radiation but without those interventions, he wouldn't have lasted 22 months and what quality of life he might have had during that period would have been severely compromised. Classic Catch 22: damned if you do and damned if you don't.

We learnt a lot in that time but they are lessons we could have done without. We didn't need to know about brain cancer, glioblastoma multiforme and dealing with the loss of a child. We are smarter now but none the wiser. Dianne gets angry and doesn't understand why bad people seem to live long and happy lives while good people die young. This is overly simplistic and her emotions are very complex and raw but if I wanted to describe her anger then I think this is not a bad characterisation. I don't get angry as it is a waste of energy to blame a situation that had no catalyst and no basis; it just happened and we dealt with it the best we could but the disease was always one step ahead. We played catch up but didn't catch anything in the end other than a whole lot of unanswered questions.

But how are we different now than we were before this started? We are the same people but we are broken. There is no easy way to explain it. Jack was our first child together and he took nearly four years to conceive (he was never in a hurry to do anything!). And he was perfect in every way, so how do you deal with that? I am sure there are a lot of psychologists out there shaking their collective heads and saying classic grieving: they need help. Yep we do, but I don't want to pay somebody to listen to me cry when I have friends and family that will do it for free.

And so this book is my way of venting, remembering, reminiscing and maybe, just maybe, I can help save a life and the universe will be in harmony again. Dianne and I would have given our life in exchange for Jack in a heartbeat but there was no place we could go to arrange such a trade. We have life and Jack doesn't, so we have to embrace what he lost and make a difference.

This is the beginning of that journey.

the beginning

THIS IS A STORY ABOUT ONE OF MY SIX SONS, THE third and the first child I had with Dianne, my wife of 22 years and my companion for 26. We called him Jack as I always wanted a Jack and didn't get my way with my first two sons.

Of six boys, two were almost perfect as toddlers and young children – Stefan and Jack. Both boys woke up each day without a cry or a whine, just happy to greet a new day and discover things. I remember Stefan just content in his cot – standing up, making sounds, sitting down, making more sounds and his face would split when he saw you, but he was never in a hurry to be set free.

Jack was content with anything and curious about everything, so self-absorbed that his parents were sidelined and took bit parts in his life, with the only intrusions for feeding and nappy changes. I think Jack would have figured everything else out as he rolled, crawled, walked and eventually ran through life.

I recall the time when he was about six months old and we took him to Noosa for a holiday. Each night we would go out

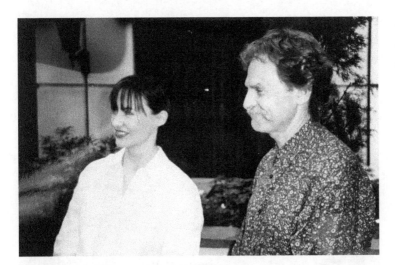

Dianne and Ken,
Melbourne,
2 March 1996

to a different restaurant and each night he would lie in his pram smiling at the world, giggling at his own private jokes or quietly absorbing his surroundings. He delighted the restaurant's staff with his quiet, no-fuss, life is cool, demeanour.

That was Jack: who needs anything else when I've got me?

Jack was born around 8 pm on 25 November 1996 at Paddington Women's Hospital in Sydney. He suffered meconium aspiration, which stopped or severely compromised his breathing, causing a mild panic in the attending medical staff. Dianne could not see the emergency play out as she was experiencing the highs of the epidural anaesthesia that had been given at the outset of labour and had her back to Jack.

I thought we were losing him as fast as we had welcomed him into the world.

Two years after Jack was born, Matthew followed and the twins (Chris and Hugh and in that order) arrived in 2000. The twins were unplanned and we have never let them forget it!

Jack and Dianne,
November 1996

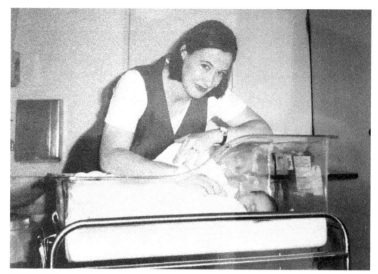

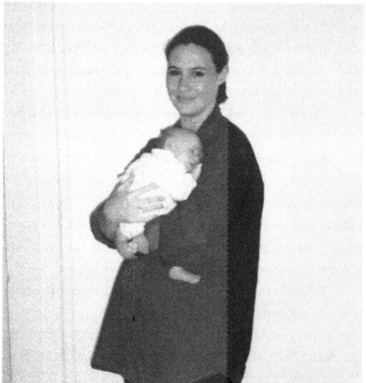

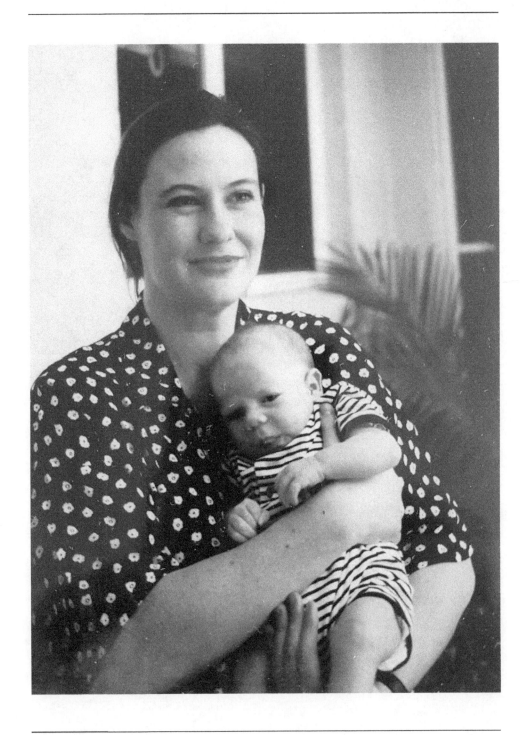

Jack and Matt, 1998

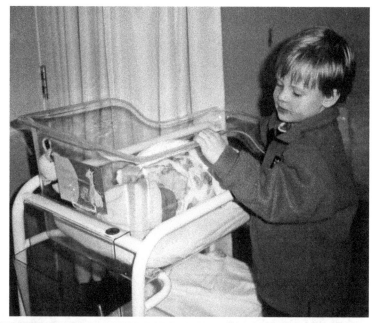

"... and when you grow up, you can become a racing car driver just like me."

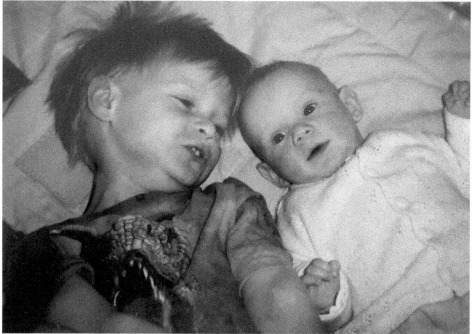

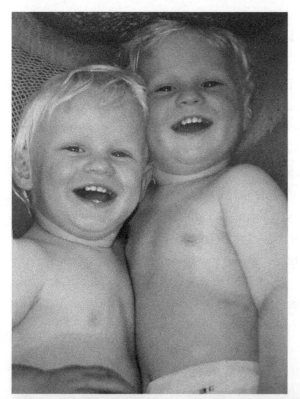

Hugh, left, and Chris, 2001

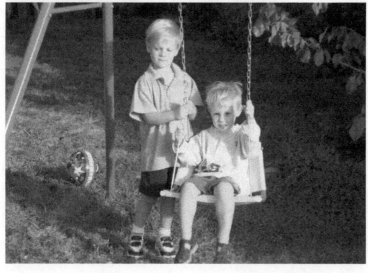

*Jack and Matt,
2001*

We were a typical (although large) "extended" family. I had two boys from a previous marriage – Stefan and Adrian. Stefan was born in 1985 and Adrian in 1990. Their mother moved from Sydney to Canberra to Bega and eventually to Hobart and every two weeks (and in some cases three weeks) I would pick the boys up on a Friday evening or Saturday morning from their home and take them to some accommodation I had arranged for the weekend and then bring them back home on Sunday afternoon. And of course, we shared the school holidays. So, life was full and Dianne and I were busy, but happy and in love.

We moved to Hobart from Sydney in 2000 after deciding that our hatred of Sydney could only be appeased by leaving the joint. We originally planned to move to Melbourne but in the end decided to continue south to be closer to my two older sons (after their mother moved to Hobart several years earlier). Dislike of Sydney was a major consideration but I was also having a mid-career crisis and questioning my ongoing commitment in a senior role at Deutsche Bank.

Dianne and I worked together for several years and were married to different people but as our marriages broke down, we found solace in each other's company and the rest, well, is history. The year was 1992 and Dianne was 27 and I was 42. We tried for several years to have a child but Dianne's plumbing needed some rewiring and when the doctors' figured that out, along came Jack. And in 1996, Dianne became a mother and her smile lit up the universe. She was complete.

Jack was an easy baby (like Stefan) but Matthew, well he was a little more normal and challenging. Dianne was spoiled by Jack, but Matthew was a reality check and he had no fear. Whereas Jack would run a full diagnostic check before he

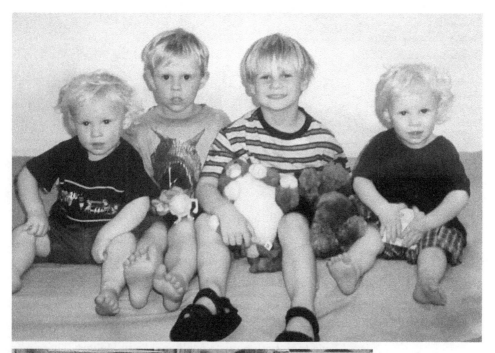

*Chris, Matt, Jack
and Hugh,
c 2001*

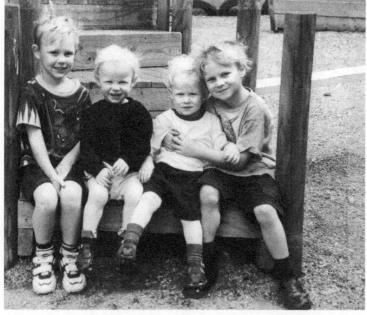

*Matt, Hugh,
Chris and Jack,
c 2002*

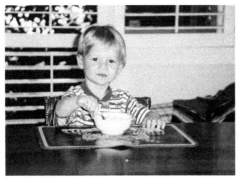 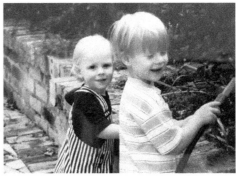

left Jack, Woolwich, Sydney, 1999

right Matt and Jack, Woolwich, c 1999.

climbed up anything or jumped anywhere, with Matthew it was always head first. Still, Jack and Matthew grew up with each other and their nightly baths together became classic blue cinema (which Matthew still hates to be reminded of and even more so to be shown the nude baby bath videos).

Several years later when Matthew would have been 5 and Jack 7, we took both boys to McDonald's in Hobart. There was a boy in the playground (maybe 6 or 7) where Jack and Matt were playing and he wasn't being nice so Jack pointed the boy out to Matthew and said, "Get him Matt". So Matt bent down like a matador and charged across the playground, bowling the boy over, flat on his back. The boy got such a shock he started crying. Jack and Matt loved that story and never got tired of hearing it. It was well ingrained in Fleming folklore and in Jack's final letter to Matt he wrote how much he loved that story.

Matt had no fear – the first in the water (no matter how cold) and the last out. Jack was the last one in the water and between him and Hugh it was a race to be the first one out. Although in Hugh's defence, he only came out when he was turning blue, which was often, as he had no fat and

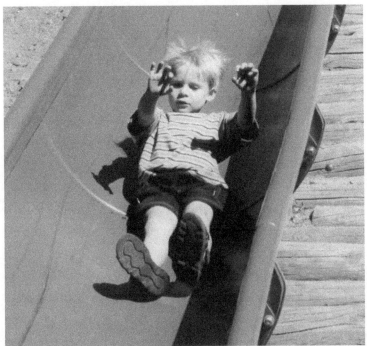

Jack, Hobart,
c 2001

Matt, left, and
Jack, learning
to swim, South
Hobart. c 2001/2

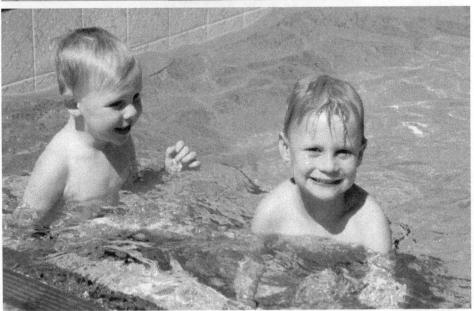

was always wafer thin. And there were many times in the chilly Tasmania water (even in summer), when this skinny little boy would run up the beach, blue and covered in goose bumps and shivering like he was fitting and barely audible, stutter "towel, towel please".

If Matthew saw a toy on an island surrounded by a moat full of sharks, electric eels, piranhas and sea snakes, he would dive in and start swimming; Jack by contrast would sit on the bank and figure out just how many minutes Matt would last before he was eaten. But there was no greater contrast between the two boys than when they were eating: Jack would pick up one noodle at a time and look at it and then put it in his mouth and chew for several minutes, while Matt would grab as much as he could in his hand and shove it into his mouth and then grab another handful while still chewing the first. And eating ice cream, Jack could eat an ice cream and his face would be spotless but Matt was lucky to get anything into his mouth and you had to give him a raincoat or give him the ice cream while he was in the bath.

When we sold the house in Woolwich in 1999 and were planning our trip to Hobart, Dianne and I decided to go to Melbourne for a dirty weekend and left Jack and Matt with family in Sydney. Nine months later Chris was born and five minutes after that out popped Hugh. Yep, identical twins! It was a disaster as I had a job that kept me interstate (Melbourne) during the week and I spent 1-2 months overseas each year while Dianne was in Hobart with no support (family or friends) and had two small boys and now the twins. The solution was nannies, as Dianne, as competent and self-sufficient as she was, could not cope.

The twins, like their older four brothers when they were little, were gorgeous. But bedtime and naptime were a nightmare as one boy would always be less tired than the other and they would then stimulate each other, eventually climbing out of their cots and wreaking havoc throughout the house until they were discovered and returned to bed. I have never hit a child and with the first four I was never tempted, but with the twins there were moments when I thought some principles *might* need to be revisited. But as they got a little older I sought my revenge through other means, such as the foot dragging episodes. When the boys were in separate beds I would tuck them in, kiss them goodnight, then turn out the light and close the door but stay in the room. I would then drag my foot across the floor walking towards them and they would go nuts! Payback boys, Daddy wins!! And they now legitimately claim this was child abuse – and by today's standards I agree.

The holidays were real adventures as each year we did a road trip to different parts of the state to explore and discover this wonderful place. And in the early years they were just young boys who played well together, swam together, chased each other around the house and bush tracks and laughed. Dianne and I also matured together; trying to understand each other a little better and accommodating nuances, quirks, likes, hates and everything in between. But I changed more than she did – I had to – as she was smarter than me, but it took me a decade to figure that out! She is far from perfect and there are aspects of her personality that I would not hesitate to change (she was born angry), although you could not find anyone more loyal, more caring, more accommodating, more supportive and conciliatory than Dianne. She is an imperfect (but beautiful) package. And we have faced chasms in our relationship that have nearly broken us but nothing like the schism we faced after Jack died: empty, broken and hollow people that could not mitigate each other's pain although we saw it, understood it and shared it.

My marriage to my second wife broke down in January 1992 but I always tried to see past the personal machinations of two angry people and focus on my two boys, Stefan and Adrian. Every second weekend I travelled from Sydney to Canberra and when they moved to Bega, I then drove from Sydney to there every fortnight (leaving Friday night and staying in Canberra and completing the trip early Saturday morning) and back home on Sunday. Bega is just over 500 km from Sydney and the drive took nearly six hours straight. I cried a lot on the way back but what could I do? The family courts were so slated towards women back then, men didn't stand a chance. Advice? Yes, I had oodles of it from marriage guidance councillors, lawyers and victims and I was in for a hiding from Hell if I tried to change the custody and access arrangements. The prejudice favouring the mother was institutionally enshrined in the psyche and manifesto of the court and the count was women 9, men 1. I hear now "things are different" but it is academic, as the time when I needed compassion and understanding the judicial system was found wanting.

opposite

top left Adrian, Thredbo, 1992

top right Adrian c 1993

bottom left Stefan, 1986

bottom right Stefan, rear, and Adrian, c 1995

And Dianne was so supportive but in the end my pain was absolute and it couldn't be cuddled or hugged away.

But I made the most of those times with the boys. I would get a unit in a motel in Tathra (16 km from Bega) and the boys would spend hours in the pool and spa, trying different tricks, splashing madly as I swam up under them and grabbed their

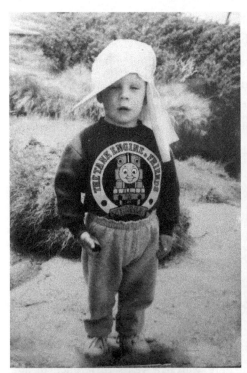
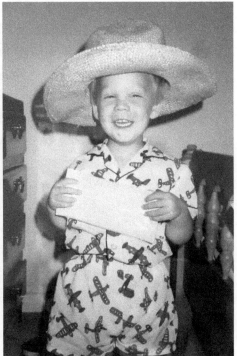
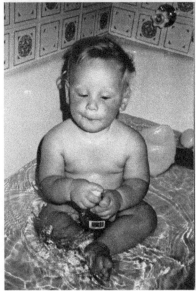
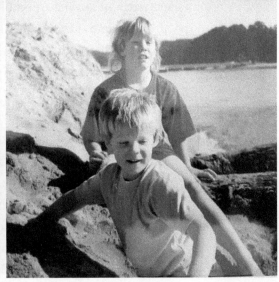

legs and perfecting the most imperfect dives. And there were the sand dunes and the rocks, which we would clamber over, climb up and down, around and across and pretend that we were on some rugged mountain range somewhere. At night I would either cook 'chicken surprise' (I can't cook so anything with chicken was the 'surprise') or we would eat in one of the local restaurants. I would also play simple mathematical games with the boys (usually using algebra) or noughts and crosses. We would play these games by scribbling on serviettes (don't know why I never thought to bring paper!). Stefan later commented that he feels the mathematical quizzes were what inspired him to have a greater interest in mathematics and eventually pursue a career as an engineer. Both boys agree, however, that chicken surprise was yet another form of child abuse.

Adrian was the spelling champion. Even when he was little he could figure out the spelling for most words (as I could when I was his age). There was five years difference in age between Stefan and Adrian but every time Stefan (or Chalkie, the nickname I gave him and still use today) got stuck on a word, he would defer to Adrian who always knew the answer. The relationship was quaintly symbiotic: Chalkie on the numbers and Adrian on the words.

When Adrian was very young, I think 2-3, he would sit on the wooden floor of our kitchen in Denistone East, Sydney, spread his legs and bang his head against the floorboards. To say we were perplexed would be a monumental understatement so we took him to the doctor. The doctor laughed and said, "Don't fret, he will stop when it starts to hurt!" And he did, eventually. He was as cute as a button and in my new-found single life, a great chick magnet: "Oh, what a cute little boy!" ... "What's your name handsome?". I recall when Dianne and I (pre-Jack) took Stefan and Adrian to the Gold Coast for a holiday and Adrian was in the pool in a tyre (he would have been 3-4 years old). He was surrounded by a group of young girls (very early teens) and they took turns pushing the tyre in a circle amongst themselves: as "he is so cute!". But Adrian wasn't happy and he was stressing and calling "Dad, Dad, Dad!!". So I rescued him from the Amazons.

When Dianne and I were plotting our escape from Sydney, we planned to move to Melbourne, however I said if we do that I will be spending every second weekend in Hobart and she said, why don't we all move to Hobart and you can commute back to Melbourne during the week and spend the weekend here? (My job with Deutsche Bank was flexible so that was doable.) So that was the plan, but on one condition: she made me agree that when I was back in Hobart that I didn't work and my weekends were all about the family.

In early January 2000, we loaded up the car, strapped Jack and Matt in and headed south. Dianne was pregnant and we didn't know it. Matt was a pain in the arse and typically challenging and I didn't know who was going to burst at the seams first – Dianne or Matt. Dianne is sometimes wound so tightly it doesn't take a lot to set her off but then again Matt wasn't happy about sitting in a baby seat for around 1,000 kilometres, so they both had some issues to work through.

Jack sat quietly, slept, giggled and chilled.

in the middle of the beginning

WELL A COUPLE OF THINGS WENT WRONG WITH the perfect plan: Dianne was pregnant with twins and I was in Melbourne or overseas and only home (on most but not all weekends) and Stefan and Adrian weren't interested in spending time with babies. They wanted to spend time with me and resented the compromise, which I get now, but back then I was a father learning to be a father and like most of us, I had big 'L' plates on.

But we muddled through and thought our life was better overall and the decision was the right one. At the end of 2000, we bought a house in Lower Sandy Bay (Nutgrove) and we were 300 metres from the beach. So on those beautiful, lazy, warm summer days over the next couple of years, we would take the boys down to the beach, lather them up with sunscreen and watch them splash, swim, wade, build sand castles and run away from me as I chased them up and down the beach. I would always have a soccer ball and we would play football on the beach. I tried to teach them how to kick and pass and tackle but it wasn't long before they were running rings around me.

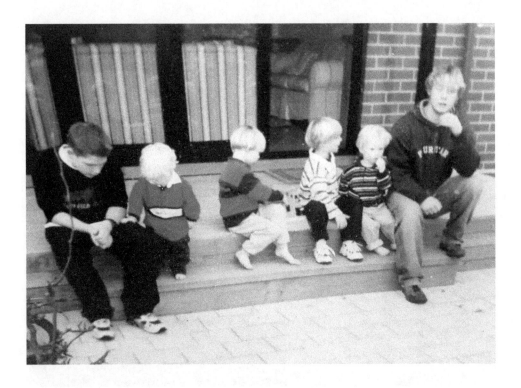

Lunch was fish and chips on the beach with soft drink (oh this is so Australian!) and then home by 1, for a hose down and afternoon nap. Saturday night was always pizza, which was a five-minute walk from the house. Same pizzas every time, with garlic bread and soft drink, and then a five-minute break to take Hugh outside while he threw up his soft drink and then back to finish the rest of the pizzas! Why we always made the same mistake regarding Hugh and his sensitive stomach defies common sense but it became a family tradition and there was plenty of dirt around the old tree just outside the restaurant door and he had his favourite spot and *whoosh*.

I think I balanced my relationship with all my boys well, but Dianne was the gem. She was born to be a mother and

*from left
Adrian, Hugh,
Matt, Jack, Chris
and Stefan*

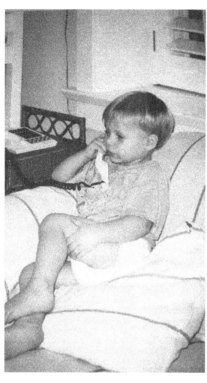
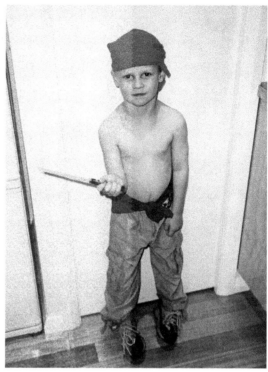

left Jack, c 1999, "Sell 5,000 BHP and buy 2000 CBA and buy me some puts on AMP!"

right Jack, c 2002

she should be awarded a Noble Prize for how she juggled my temperament, endless nappy changes, meals, the twins' eczema, baths and bedtime stories. It is beyond my comprehension but you knew she always had her shit together. And she was a little crazy – balancing her naturally combative personality with the chaos and satisfaction of being a mother of four dynamic, gorgeous, funny young men. Interesting juxtaposition that one.

Midway through 2002, Deutsche and I parted ways and that introduced some new challenges.

In 2003, we moved to Lenah Valley and into a beautiful old 2.5 storey house on 2,000 square metres of land. It is memorable for its aesthetics, charm, a nutty neighbour and the near death of

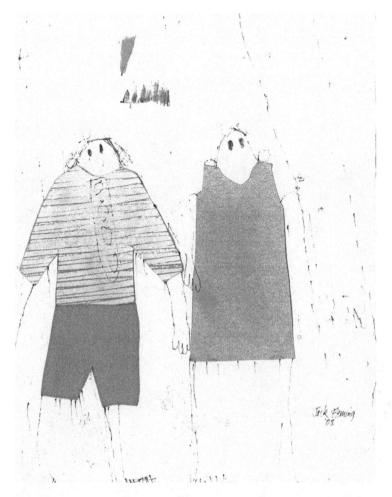

Drawing by Jack, 2003

the twins, as well as the fact that we never realised how much the house meant to Jack until we left it. He loved the house, he told us after we sold it, and missed it a lot. And I have thought many times since whether that acute sense of loss was the catalyst for the tumour in his brain, which eventually took his life. Then again I had a million theories and not one mattered then and even less now as fate's hand has been dealt.

Jack's story

Hugh, Jack, Matt and Chris, Lenah Valley, c 2005

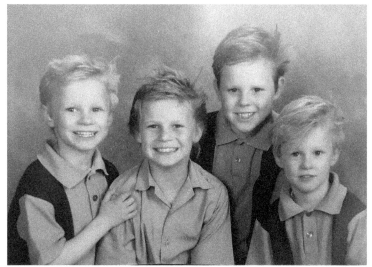

Matt, Jack, Chris and Hugh, Lenah Valley, c 2007

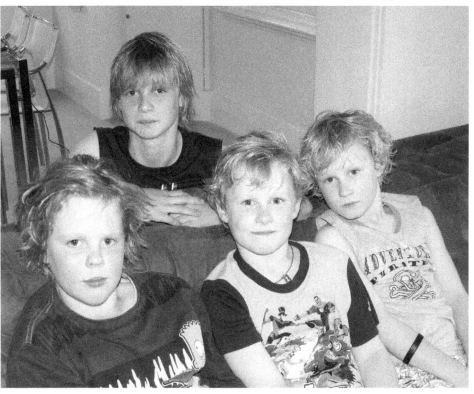

The situation with the twins was a moment of truth for Dianne and I and was the closest we had ever come, at least at that time, to losing a child (and in this case two children). Because we had four young boys and a large property we would check on everyone every hour or so if we didn't know where they were. You could never let your guard down unless you knew they were tucked up in bed and asleep. There was this one time that I had returned from a trip interstate and the twins came into the lounge room where I was sitting and asked for my car keys. I said I didn't have them but that they were probably in the kitchen somewhere. It was summer and warm outside and I think I dosed, only woken by Dianne asking me where were the twins. I completely forgot that they had asked for the car keys and said they were here a little while ago but I haven't seen them since. No panic, just the usual checks and balances and rollcall.

So, we split up and went through the house thinking they were hiding. This would have been 2003 or 2004 so the twins were 3 or 4. We looked all around the backyard, but there was no sign of them. Dianne started to panic and thought they may have gone out the front and walked up the street and/or even been abducted. She often opined they would be kidnapped because they were so cute. For Dianne this was a real and ever-present worry and she was beginning to think that fear was now a reality. This fuelled my own growing feeling of panic and we both rushed outside and Dianne started to walk up the street calling out their names. Nothing. But then Dianne heard a very faint voice and it came from the boot of the car. As she screamed for me to open the boot it hit me that they had asked for my car keys and that is where they would be! How we got

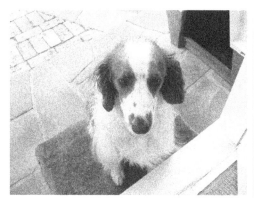 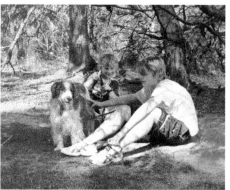

left Lola

right Lola, Hugh
and Matt, c 2007

the boot open I don't recall but it was either the spare set of keys or the car was open (and the boot latch is under the dashboard).

When we opened the boot, Hugh was nearly asleep and Chris barely conscious and they were both dripping wet. Another 10 minutes they would have fallen asleep and baked to death if we hadn't found them because we would never have thought about the looking in the car boot. So many tears, but tears of joy and relief. They had climbed in there looking for the two plastic swords that we had bought them some time ago and one of them had the bright idea to close the boot while they were inside.

Lola joined us around 2006. She was an interesting inclusion in our family life as I didn't want a dog but Dianne insisted and one day she bought Lola home – pedigree Welsh Springer Spaniel. I ignored her for the first 12 months but she had the most beautiful temperament and eventually I succumbed to her canine charms. One rule I insisted on however was that she was not allowed inside the house. Well that was good for a day because as soon as Dad was away from the house, in came Lola. Dianne was #2 culprit but Jack was an unequivocal #1. Jack and Lola had a special bond and he spent more time with her than any of the other boys and increasingly so, the sicker they both got.

Football (with the round ball) was our passion and Stefan played it at school and on weekends, as did Jack, Chris, Adrian and Hugh. Matt on the other hand tried it but he was not interested in sport (more interested in eating!). And we had our English Premier League teams – I was Liverpool, Hugh Chelsea and Jack, Chris and Adrian were Arsenal. Neither Matt nor Stefan had a team. And this rivalry defined many conversations and mealtime arguments as the boys grew up and our positions became more entrenched and our impassioned defences more vocal.

ARSENAL FC

Arsenal, like Liverpool, had so many lost opportunities that Jack was (particularly in this last year of his life) perpetually frustrated. However, his #2 team was Liverpool so he enjoyed the highs (and sometimes the lows) of Liverpool's season as well.

Ironically, Jack (with about 20 friends) set up a fantasy football team whereby the players you have in the team are awarded points after each match they play in for their real team. The EPL finished the week beginning 15 May 2018 – and Jack came first!! He had been dead for exactly one month.

He would have been chuffed.

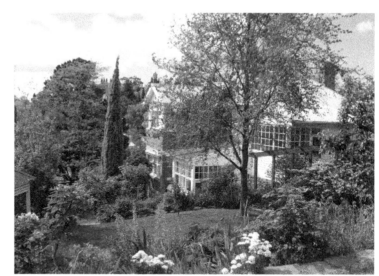

*Our house in
Lenah Valley*

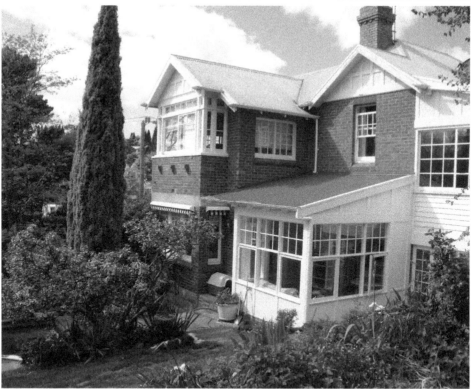

Adrian's interest in playing football was, however, marginal while Stefan confined his passion to his school team where in his final year (Year 10 as he was over school after that) his first-grade team won the inter-school competition undefeated. But in Jack in those early days we recognised his raw talent and speed on the field and a star was born (at least in my eyes). So I would watch Jack's games and Dianne would watch the twins' games (but they were so young back then it was a melee with feet, legs and arms going in any direction the ball was moving and many times in any direction). If the times didn't clash I would also get to see the twins playing (they were so cute but hopeless). But they matured and as the years rolled on and Jack was forced to stop playing after his first seizure, I would watch the twins and they developed into solid and highly skilled footballers. Jack used to say they were "shit" (jokingly) but after the few games he watched and after he was diagnosed with GBM, he conceded that they were so much better than him. I wouldn't agree but to be diplomatic, I would say on a par.

And there was also futsal, which became more significant in our lives as Jack's disease progressed.

Futsal is indoor soccer and I am sure the extremists would know the difference but to me it is soccer, played indoors, on a basketball court and with the same frenetic pace as basketball. Adrian played it as did Stefan (although he would refer to it as 'indoor soccer') but Jack and the twins grew into it and unlike their older brothers, played it for many years. The twins were always in the same team and Jack played with a team with older players. And fuck they were good! So exciting to watch. I would usually always manage to get to both games and they collectively won a lot of competitions.

So with futsal, soccer, training, water polo, underwater hockey (yes it exists), tennis, school and discovery holidays, and time spent with Adrian and Stefan, life was pretty full and probably on balance pretty normal (if of course you think six boys is normal).

We moved to Tranmere around 2009 as a result of the GFC. While our house in Lenah Valley was our home and over nearly 2,000 square metres provided plenty of space for the boys and Lola to run and for Dianne to plant many fruit trees, it was not practical as we had a liquidity crunch. We rented in Tranmere for nearly two years and eventually bought the house we were renting. Dianne did not want to buy the house as she thought it was ugly and she couldn't do much to improve its bones. However, I prevailed on the basis that the price was right; the footprint was nearly 40 squares and offered five bedrooms and three bathrooms; land size was 800 square metres; we had panoramic views of the water and were two-minute walk away from the river; 20 minutes into the city in peak hour; it was quite and we had great neighbours! And the neighbours in particular were wonderful and rallied behind us when they found out about Jack and supported the family right to the end.

Jack

JACK WAS A QUIET ACHIEVER – ALWAYS DID VERY well at school, sport and particularly chess. However, when he was around 6, it was discovered that he was nearly deaf and after that he wore two hearing aids. He said that defined a lot of his character at school as he didn't understand most of the jokes (as he didn't hear them) and thus it was sometimes difficult to respond. He became very shy and reserved and blamed those traits on his hearing loss and fear of speaking out of context because he missed the cue.

He also exploited it and referred to himself as the "disabled one" and when Dianne was on his case he sometimes turned his hearing aids off and said loudly, "I can't hear you!". He also used to joke as his brain became more addled from the cancer and treatments, and he lost a lot of his sight from one of the drugs we introduced – ABT414 – that he was becoming deaf, dumb and blind. Each week he set a reminder to change the batteries and even now, several months after his death, the message still comes up on his phone (we check his phone each day for Facebook messages and memories).

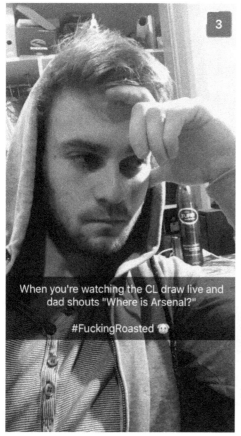

When you're watching the CL draw live and dad shouts "Where is Arsenal?"

#FuckingRoasted 💀

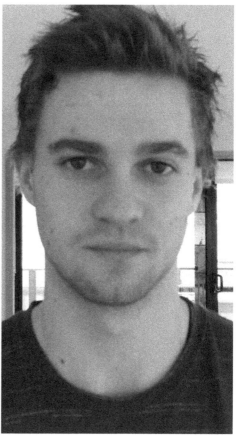

He didn't ask too many questions but when he did he was never frustrated if he didn't get the answer he wanted as he knew he would always figure something out. And he did.

I wonder as I write this, just how do you encapsulate the essence of a person in a word, phrase or sentence so that people who didn't know Jack will start to nod and say, 'I get it'. Probably the best example that I can refer to is when he was in pre-school, at Lady Gowrie in Battery Point. His teachers adored him as he was such as easy child but he tended to play by himself. When we would pick him up in the afternoon, he would always be sitting in a corner, crossed leg with a puzzle and fully absorbed in what he was doing. As he sensed your presence he would look up and smile, "Oh it is time to go home already?" as he stood up and took your hand.

If Jack saw someone with a toy that he wanted he would wait until the child became bored with it and walked away. Now take Matt, he was a force to be reckoned with at Lady Gowrie because if he saw a toy, and regardless if someone had it or not and he wanted it, he would take it. Matt was always in a hurry; Jack sedentary by comparison.

Occasionally when he was younger he would sleepwalk and typically when asked about it the following day, not remember a thing. Once I kissed him on the forehead – as I did with all the boys as I did the rounds to make sure everyone was soundly asleep – and he opened his eyes and said to me: "What are you doing going around and kissing boys at night!?". 'Wow,' I thought, 'where did that come from?' Heavy, heavy. But of course, he never remembered it.

As he got older and went through puberty, he became very insular and getting answers to the most basic questions became challenging. Prior to his diagnosis, we would get the most perfunctory response to general questions, like:

"Where did you go last night?"

"Out.

"I know that, but where to, a bar?"

"Yes."

"Which bar?"

"In town and why do you ask me so many questions!?"

And so it went.

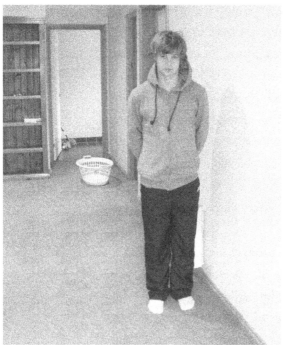
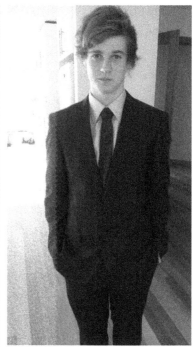

left Jack,
c 2012/14

right Jack
dressed for his
school formal,
2014

He didn't bring friends home although he was always out with friends. We often quizzed him about a girlfriend but he would typically clam up, smile and walk away. The irony is that we really only started to know the mature Jack after he was diagnosed and became increasingly fragile and vulnerable. But there was always a quiet charm in the room when Jack was there and you couldn't help but feel the strength of his personality, and his quiet, but powerful, presence. And he had the unequivocal respect and adulation of his younger brothers. His older brothers were distant when he was growing up due to the different family circumstances but in the last five years became a lot closer and it started to feel like the one big family with six siblings. Stefan and

Adrian became very close to Jack after he was diagnosed and the many times they visited after July 2016 it was all about Jack and he was never alone.

But Jack was a contentious character as well, as he was so competitive and the many squabbles that the boys were engaged in were usually at the provocation of Jack who would bait everyone regarding school, computer game prowess, height, bench pressing, haircuts, friends and football. Yet in one area he was clearly better than anyone else and that was chess. When I was growing up there was no TV, computers, Facebook or mobile phones, so board games dominated our play time. I was never a passionate chess player and would suggest my track record could be, at best, described as 'average'. Jack, however, was a natural and that characterised a lot about Jack as he was good at no matter what he applied himself to and particularly his studies.

When he went to university he was unsure of what he would like to do but settled on Law and Business (with a major in Finance). He won the Australian Stock Market challenge for Tasmania in his final year at school and thought maybe he would follow in my footsteps. And although he excelled in all his studies – high distinctions and distinctions for all his subjects – he was never really sure of what he wanted to be at the end. I didn't really care as he had the intelligence and academic smarts that he could do whatever he wanted to do. Moreover, he was a handsome young man and a natural sportsman and, dare I say, the full package?

Matthew, I think, sometimes felt jaded and often opined to Dianne that, "He is the golden hair boy!". And yes, maybe we did lay it on too thick but besides his hearing, Jack was hands-free. But as I look back now, and since his death, I wonder if I missed some things, as from the collation of comments from one of his ex-teachers and some of the old photos, I now see a boy that was not always happy and was, at times, very distracted and, I think, troubled?

How did I miss that? I just always thought Jack had it all together, so I concentrated my pastoral care activities on his other five brothers. Stefan and Adrian had odd choices for girlfriends in their youth and there were the inevitable stress points and fatherly intervention but they lived with their mother and I was (sometimes), an unwanted distraction. Matthew was a big boy and bullied in primary school (which we fixed by moving him to Friends) but I would try and sit with him as often as possible and see how he was travelling. And he was very open (unlike Jack who told you jack shit!) and spoke freely and always from the heart (which he regularly wore on his sleeve). The twins? Well they were off and running and had each other and developed very robust and engaging personalities but as they got older there were times when I would pick up a subtle change in their demeanour and ask them directly if everything was OK.

Jack had a very special relationship with Dianne and I used to say (and meant it) Dianne was his favourite. I felt no jealousy or bitterness about this and was actually flattered that Jack recognised in Dianne the same characteristics that made me fall in love with her so many years earlier. But more important than this was the strength of our relationship to Jack and I would sometimes see out of the corner of my eye Jack's face whenever Dianne and I showed each other affection. He would be watching unashamedly and smiling. In that relationship, Jack saw security and harmony and if that relationship was ever threatened Jack would blame me, no matter the circumstances. For instance, if Dianne and I had a disagreement and I was somewhere with Jack and venting, he would become angry with me and tell me I was wrong. Even if Dianne stuck a knife in my face, garrotted me and burnt my body in the backyard and scattered my ashes to the wind, Jack would still have blamed me. And while I could have an objective discussion with the other three boys about their mother, any criticism of Dianne to Jack was met with a rush of anger and a quick retort. Even when I was defending him! So I learnt to never say anything negative (no matter how balanced) about Dianne to Jack, and I kept my own counsel on Dianne to myself whenever Jack was in earshot.

I used to joke with Dianne (although there was some seriousness to my suggestion) that Jack would never leave home, as he was so happy here: he had his own room, his family, his clothes washed, meals cooked and security. He was content; between study, work at the Lark Distillery at Cambridge and his friends, he didn't worry about making time for anything else.

But even as he became more aloof as he crashed through puberty and finished high school, we always had one passion in common (other than football) and that was whisky. He worked at the Lark Whisky Bar in Hobart and later at the distillery at Cambridge. And as his illness advanced, that comradery and job became increasingly important to him even when we thought it best that he didn't go to work on some days. However, he persevered until it was impossible to continue working. Still he would always have a whisky or two with me and discuss what he thought the nose and palate revealed.

My passion for whisky went beyond the palate and extended to the balance sheet. I have invested a significant amount of money in Lark and now, its new owner, Australian Whisky Holdings. But since Jack was diagnosed, a couple of my fellow whisky tragics and I decided to set up our own company – Elmside Single Malt – and I asked Jack to become an investor. He was stoked and took 10% of the company. My thinking was several fold: it would be a welcome distraction for him; it might (when the whisky matures and we start to sell it after 5-6 years) make a lot of money; but my overriding reason was that it could give him a job if we were successful and he survived the cancer.

And Jack had money. He never spent anything and all those years working for Lark he saved every penny. In addition, and more significantly, he claimed full settlement of his life insurance on the grounds of his terminal illness. The background to this claim was unusual, as neither I (nor Jack nor Dianne) knew he had life insurance and I only discovered it after he was being treated and I was looking through his superannuation fund statement. I rang the fund and asked for a copy of the policy and when I read it I found the "early payment" in event of terminal illness clause. All we had to do was establish that he was going to die. Well that seemed easy but as I spoke to his clinicians to get the paperwork completed, the weight of what I was establishing buried me. They were only pieces of paper but in those papers were sentences stating that Jack Fleming had an incurable and terminal disease and had only a short time to live. And my job was to prosecute that argument and establish beyond reasonable doubt he was dying.

CRYING
the unavoidable reality

Never did much (or any?) crying growing up but my earlier adult years were marked by the untimely deaths of two very good friends – my brother-in-law, John and my very dear friend Ron. John died of non-Hodgkin's lymphoma in 1992 and Ron died of primary bowel cancer in 2003, which, typically spread to all his vital organs.

I can never recall hearing myself cry until the day Johnny passed. I remember walking back to the underground car park at the hospital and then heard this wailing that broke uncontrollably from me as I made my way to my car – that deep sense of loss, despair and unquenchable sadness that most of us have felt at some point in our lives. And with Ron, the same. But the dam really broke when I, as one of the pallbearers, carried his coffin to the hearse. And the weight. He was around 6' 6" and while not overweight, I remember feeling acutely conscious that this is all that is left of my dear friend and he was so, so heavy.

With Jack, crying (and sometimes howling) became a daily (and hourly) occurrence and even in conversations with people I barely knew, the voice started to crack, and the words dried up and the tears jammed my eyes. Dianne and I cried so often we stopped trying to comfort each other, as two souls in pain had nothing to give the other person other than more pain. But there were highs when one of us made a discovery or spoke to a person that offered hope, and sometimes there were tears of joy and not despair as we convinced ourselves and/or each other we had a pathway.

But every pathway and every rabbit hole made no difference to the outcome. We might have gained days, weeks or even months and then again, we may have lost days, weeks and months through the course we were advised to follow and that, ultimately was our decision, we agreed to follow.

EARLIER HEALTH HISTORY

Jack's health had been robust his entire life until he was diagnosed with brain cancer. We thought about this a lot, looking for the "trigger" for what he was diagnosed with on 8 July 2016, but other than X-rays and MRIs for his braces, there was nothing. Some of the literature on brain cancer has pointed to X-rays and MRIs of the head as possible causes but, like mobile phone usage, the causal link has never been unequivocally established. And why doesn't every child who has braces and requires X-rays and/or MRIs get brain cancer?

So, there were no answers and this is typical of most people who get brain cancer: shit happens.

This is it in a nutshell:

1   Hearing: diagnosed with a mild to moderate sensorineural hearing loss in both ears at age 6. He wore hearing aids routinely ever since. Over time, there was deterioration in hearing thresholds, particularly in the right ear. At the time of his cancer diagnosis, his audiogram showed mild to moderately severe hearing loss in his left ear, and severe loss in the right.

2   Compartment syndrome: both calves; severe pain and loss of sensation in both feet even after walking the dog for 20 minutes. Jack suffered for almost two years before an operation on 1 December 2014 on all four compartments. This was very successful with no complications, and he was able to return to playing soccer and gym in February the next year.

3   Braces: top and bottom.

His hearing problem was a frustration for everyone, including of course Jack, as you had to look at him directly and raise your voice. I found sometimes when he was growing up that when I was trying to explain some more complex issues I would get exhausted, as it is not easy to think quickly and then speak slowly at a decibel or two above your normal level. And unless he wore his special headphones, the TV had to be turned up to a level that was uncomfortable for my ears. So life with Jack was challenging at times.

But the compartment syndrome problem possibly frustrated him more as he couldn't play football and if he did manage to get off the bench, he was back on it within 20 minutes. And football was his (and my) life so I shared his frustration. In 2016, he joined Clarence United and started as a full back, an odd position for Jack who was usually the fastest person on the team and always played as a forward. I asked him why he accepted that position and not up front and he just shrugged his shoulders and said he was happy at the back. Well I reckon he stayed there for one, maybe two games as when they realised how quick he was they put him on the wing and he started to score goals. I remember standing on the sidelines with a couple of Clarence supporters that did not know him and I heard one say: "Who is that?".

He pointed at Jack and his mate said, "Jack Fleming".

"Wow he is fast; great legs".

After his first seizure in May that year, he never played football again.

UNIVERSITY

University was a breeze, but Jack worked far too hard. His marks reflected his natural intelligence and work ethic. He flew through first year Law and Business/Economics/Finance, with finance and econometrics his favourite subjects. He loved the maths. First semester in his second year started well and then he had a seizure which put a full stop to everything. He later managed to sit his exams in Law and other subjects but post the seizure found it difficult to concentrate on Investment Analysis and even though the university was aware of his illness, failed him in that unit. I spoke to several of the Professors at the Uni that I knew, and they said that this was ridiculous as he was cruising through the subject and they had no doubt he would have achieved a High Distinction (HD).

He was belatedly awarded a HD and he said that is what he deserved anyway as he had no doubt he would have scored a HD. He could be a real arrogant smartarse sometimes.

In 2017, we got him back to Uni in the second semester, but his cognitive abilities were highly compromised; his eyesight was weak, and his short-term memory was poor and it soon became clear that he could not continue. I had pushed him to go back to Uni as I thought we would beat this thing and he would need a career. However, it became obvious to me after a while that he was not coping, and I agreed, and fully supported, his decision to quit.

Looking back now, six months after Jack died, and reading this it reminded me of that difficult juxtaposition I was forever confronted with between accepting the fact that he was going die but inwardly hoping there was a miracle due the family and he would pull through. I recall now so strongly that feeling that if he could finish university – somehow – and we – somehow – could save him, life would go on almost as if this event never happened. And I said this over and over in my head and to anyone who would listen (voluntarily or reluctantly).

the end of the beginning

STEFAN MOVED TO SYDNEY WITH HIS ENGINEERING
company and then eventually moved to Perth and started and
completed a degree in Civil Engineering. Jack kept saying to
me you must be so proud of him and of course I was as there
were moments I thought he had a greater propensity for prison
than university.

He was in a good place and was completing his degree in
Perth when Jack was diagnosed.

Adrian is a very different kettle of fish and didn't
do well in his final year (12) of school because he wasn't
interested. When he split with his then girlfriend around 2008
it was obvious that he was not in a good place and Stefan
and I decided to get him out of Tasmania and we arranged
for him to move to Sydney. He moved in with Stefan and his
then girlfriend and I got him a job with his cousin in a bar in
Sydney. And even today, at the age of 28, he is still working in
bars and loving it. Find something you are good at it and stick
to it and that speaks volumes about Adrian and his singular
career choice.

He had just started a new relationship with a French girl ("Frenchie" he calls her; we call her Ingrid) and was working happily in Melbourne when Jack was diagnosed.

Matthew is a gentle giant (at 6'2") and has the most beautiful eyes. He is however a work-in-progress as he is very sensitive and the more emotional of all my boys. So, I spent as much time with him as I could to make sure that those small hurdles, which sometimes consumed him, were addressed. He always knew he could have an open and honest conversation with me. Mathematics is his passion and he did very well in his year 12 exams and is now in his second year at university, studying mathematics and science. He plays games with his friends online at night and attends university during the day and occasionally he raids my whisky stash and depletes my stocks of Japanese malts and American rye whiskies. Plus, some of my IPAs and Dubbels (a beautiful Belgian beer). When, as more often than not, dinner conversations drifted into the hallowed ground of the English Premier League, Matt is sidelined as he cannot add anything to the conversation. And that is the way it has always been and the way it will probably always be.

But he was halfway through his Year 12 when Jack was diagnosed. And of all my boys, Dianne and I were more concerned with Matthew as this was a watershed year and we wanted nothing to distract him.

"By the way Matt, Jack has 12 months to live but don't let this stop you from getting top marks this year, OK?"

Other than nearly losing Chris and Hugh in the boot of a car when they were toddlers, they haven't missed a beat and life has treated them well. They always had each other and while there was some frosting in their relationship as they went through puberty, Jack's diagnosis and the march of time, put them back in the womb.

There have been times over the years that Dianne and I have confused them, however they have developed two distinct personalities – Hugh is like his mum and combative whereas Chris is a little more chilled. Chris is left-handed and hugs without hesitation whereas Hugh is right-handed and avoids touching.

They were in Year 10 at Friends (where Matthew was finishing Year 12 and where Jack also graduated from in 2014) when Jack was diagnosed.

And we were cruising, literally at 36,000 feet, just before the shit hit the fan. Dianne, the four boys and I went on a holiday to Hong Kong, skiing in the north of Japan and then spent a couple of days in Kyoto. It was January 2016. Adrian joined us in Hong Kong and then flew with us to Japan and spent the week teaching the boys how to use a snowboard. It was magic and the boys had a ball. Jack, Chris and Hugh had never been overseas and Matt had only spent a couple of days in New Zealand with his underwater hockey (yes, it is a real sport) team. Jack didn't complain and neither did Adrian (he is a seasoned traveller) but Matt and the twins never stopped complaining about the food and the uncomfortable seats. I thought, wow, first time overseas and I have to put up with this shit?! Wow. And I am paying for it?! But the skiing made up for everything and despite the debilitating injury to Hugh's thigh muscle, the gaping gash that needed stitches running up Jack's leg from a collision with Chris, and an earthquake, the holiday ranked alongside Hamilton Island and a couple of our early Bicheno holidays.

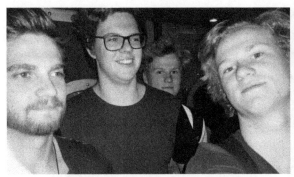 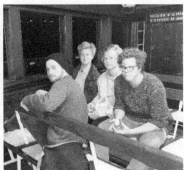

When we got back we started to plan Christmas in New York at the end of the year. We were in a good place and I remember walking early one morning (as I exercise most mornings) and thinking how good life was at the time. What could go wrong?

left Jack, Matt, Chris and Hugh, Hong Kong, January 2016

right Jack, Chris, Hugh and Matt aboard the Star Ferry, January 2016

Our life came to a screeching halt on the bitterly cold afternoon of 8 July 2016. Many parents reading this who have lost a child (or are expecting to lose a child) understand only too well that feeling of loss. Parenting is about changing nappies, spoon-feeding bowls of baby gruel, kissing elbows and reading stories as little eyes flutter and finally shut. It is guiding our children through school, first loves, career choices and everything in between. As they get older we become less relevant and that is the way it is supposed to be but sitting your son down and explaining that he doesn't have long to live because he didn't (want to) understand what the neurosurgeon had just told him and mummy and daddy can't fix this one, is a dark place no one should ever have to inhabit. But we did. Even then it didn't sink in and on the following night, he came upstairs from his bedroom where he had been for most of the day.

"Do you mean I will never finish university, go overseas, work in New York or London, get married and have children?"

"Yes," I said, it means all those things".

At that point it sank in; he got it; understood. He turned around and left the room. I cried and cried and cried.

And there were many more conversations like that, which had the same dark undertone – getting a list of all his passwords (we didn't ask for them; he just handed Dianne and I a sheet of paper one day with everything listed), preparing his will, relating the discussion with his neurosurgeon after his second surgery which confirmed he had but six months to live and discussing the results of the 17 December 2016 MRI which showed significant "enhancement" of his tumour. The latter event confirming we were close to the end and there was little else to try.

Tears don't cut it. They are the culmination of human anguish and, in many cases, heartache, but when you stop crying the problem is unchanged. Many times, I said to anyone who would listen and mainly to myself, "I will not bury my son, not now, not ever. I WILL NOT BURY MY SON!".

Over the weeks and months, that lament changed to, "I will bury my son if I have to and we, as a family, will stand strong and united". Oh such brave words, from someone who felt anything but brave.

So much promise, so much life, so much intelligence. All to be eroded and destroyed by a disease that does not discriminate by age, race or gender. It takes no prisoners. It is like watching someone with Alzheimer's – forgetful, struggling to comprehend words, let alone sentences. It re-minded me of when Jack was 4 or 5 (not 21)! – what's this word mean?; what does this mean?; can you read that to me?; do I know that word? "Pizza, pizza? I know what that is, what does it look like?"

And there were so many times, when no one was looking, I would grab the tumour in my hands and wrestle with it to the floor, stamp on it and choke it to death. I would eat it, crush it, smother it, destroy it.

A slow march into hell, but tempered by lighter moments and moments when he was very lucid, and the old Jack peeped out from under the clouds. Near the end he still believed, in his fragile state, that we were winning. But when I finally forced myself to embrace the truth, that there was no way back, he was too vulnerable to understand the implications so we continued the charade to the end.

I never got the chance to say goodbye until it was too late and he was beyond comprehension.

2016: the start

ON FRIDAY 27 MAY 2016, JACK PLAYED FOOTBALL (soccer) at King George V Oval at Glenorchy; kick off was at 7 pm. It was a cold evening and I was sitting on my own in the clubhouse, where the view was not the best but the difference in temperature made it a worthwhile compromise. Sometimes Dianne would join me and sometimes not. But it didn't matter, as I was there to watch Jack play which I always enjoyed – although if I ever criticised his performance he could get very prickly.

He played very well on the right wing and typically was one of the fastest boys on the field. I remember going over the game many times in the next couple of weeks trying to recall if any clashes or tackles he had were particularly brutal and whether he took a bad knock to the head. There was nothing I could identify so the catalyst for what transpired on the following evening was, for several weeks anyway, a complete mystery.

That evening he drove home (I had driven there separately) and we later talked about the game. I was very complimentary, as he had played very well. He had a couple of beers and went to bed. That was the last normal day of his life.

It was a typical Saturday for Dianne and I – vacuuming, gardening, washing clothes, making meals for the four boys and washing up after each meal. It was uneventful for Jack also at least until early evening when he complained of a headache. Dianne told him to take a couple of Panadol and lie down. We didn't think anything of it other than it was a little unusual, as Jack never complained of headaches.

I went to our bathroom – which has a common wall with Jack's bedroom – and heard very heavy breathing that I initially thought was snoring coming from Jack's room. Again, this was unusual, and although Jack had a penchant (albeit very rare) for sleepwalking, we don't recall ever hearing him snore. I went to the door and the sound was like very heavy breathing or snorting so if it was snoring, Jack had created his own unique sound – a bit like the sound of wood being sawn. I got Dianne from upstairs and brought her down to Jack's door. "Listen to this." She put her ear to the door then quickly opened it and we both went in. She turned on the light. Jack was slumped across his bed, his head on the floor. His breathing was very laboured, and he was dribbling. Dianne pulled him up into a sitting position against the wall, but he was not with us. His eyes were glazed and unfocused and he did not recognise anything or anybody. Dianne kept calling his name, and although he tried to speak, he could only make guttural sounds.

I know now that we were witnessing a seizure (which has a name "grand mal" seizure) but at the time we were ignorant.

The ambulance arrived 45 minutes later. Jack was out of his comatose state but far from normal; he had no understanding of what had just taken place and couldn't remember anything from the time he took the Panadol to the moment the paramedics arrived. The paramedics asked all the usual questions re drugs, medications, alcohol, history etc. and conjectured that he had had a fit or even a seizure. Jack was groggy and struggled to comprehend and answer the questions.

Dianne and I were in a state of mild shock but we were not particularly concerned as no one in the family had had any major medical conditions, so we just thought the usual – dehydrated, knock the night before at football (concussion?), allergic reaction to something?

I went with him in the ambulance and within an hour of arriving he was back to normal but had no recollection of what had taken place over the previous two hours. He was laughing and joking and more concerned with checking his phone than trying to comprehend what had put him in a bed in Emergency on a Saturday night.

Dianne later picked me up, as we thought, on advice, that we should leave him in overnight – a decision we would be forced to make on many more occasions and under more stressful and traumatic conditions.

We went to our favourite Indian restaurant, ordered some chicken tikka and a couple of naans and discussed the events of the last three hours. I sipped on some red wine and Dianne drank water. We convinced ourselves that there were a number of natural explanations – all obviously innocent – and this night would pass and never be repeated. We both slept well that night.

the next couple of weeks The clinicians were perplexed and had a number of theories, including (and principally) that it was a heart issue, so the focus was on seeing a cardiologist and undertaking a cardiogram. As we were in the 'public hospital system' – a place that was totally alien to us – we were in a queue for these tests to be undertaken, including (again no urgency) seeing a neurologist and having an MRI. Once the cardiogram showed no abnormalities, there was a heightened concern that Jack should see the neurologist as quickly as possible. The scan revealed a cloud on his brain – suspected to be a tumour – but we were assured it was not uncommon and most likely "benign". He was admitted to Calvary Hospital on 5 July for a biopsy to be undertaken by his (now) neurosurgeon, Andrew Hunn, the following day.

In the interim, Jack had stopped driving and returned to university. His licence was automatically suspended following his seizure and would not be reinstated unless he was given the all clear by a neurologist after at least three months. This loss of freedom was brutal for him but typically, he just accepted it without too much protest.

We also had to learn to navigate the health system – both private and public. We had private health cover and knew the outgoings would be minimal – little or nothing from involvement with the public system and capped when assessing the private system. Looking back and now six months since Jack died, our overall medical expenses were minimal (largely hospital bed excess of $200 no matter how long Jack was in hospital, MRIs, surgery costs and prescriptions). The chemotherapy drugs were free, except for Avastin which we threw in at the end as a last-ditch effort to make something good come from something that was turning to shit.

JULY

On Sunday 3 July, before we started our march into hell, we decided to have a long (yum cha) lunch at Me Wah Chinese restaurant in Sandy Bay.

3 July

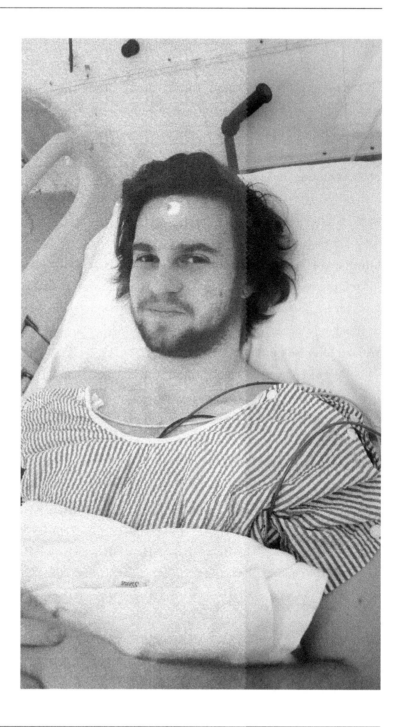

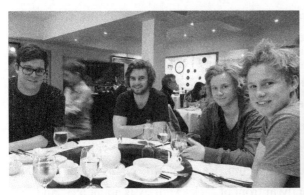 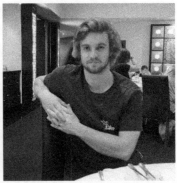

There was no reason other than we thought, why not?

Purely a bonding session with some nice food and innocent conversation, although a dark cloud was never far from the horizon and the inert fear that this could end badly was never far from the surface.

The boys were in good spirits (Stefan and Adrian were interstate, so it was Jack, Matthew, and the twins, Chris and Hugh, Dianne and I).

left Matt, Jack, Hugh and Chris at Me Wah

right Jack

We were called to a meeting at Andrew Hunn's office on Friday 8 July at 5 pm. We were light headed and in good spirits, as we had convinced ourselves that the tumour was benign. I had even booked a restaurant in North Hobart for dinner that evening in anticipation of a celebration. And in hindsight, we had every reason to be relaxed as our mutual family history was clear of any major diseases and other than several broken arms and a couple of cracked ribs: the boys were Teflon coated. Naively we also held the view that most things can be fixed through surgery, drugs or lifestyle and kids do not die of cancer (other than leukemia). And who had

8 July
5.00 pm

heard of brain cancer? Well yeah, we had but then again we had also heard of the American Civil War and the Spanish Inquisition and we knew more about those events than we did about brain cancer.

However, Andrew's demeanour was sombre, and while Dianne insisted on standing, he insisted she sit. Something was wrong. My pulse quickened. He asked Jack to sit close to his desk and nearest to him. He pulled his chair around the table and sat directly in front of Jack. Andrew is about 6' 3" and Jack 5' 9" and Andrew leant into him and spoke softly but fluently. The BOMBSHELL.

"I am afraid I have bad news for you, Jack, and wish there was some other way to tell you, but you have brain cancer and it's terminal. It's called glioblastoma multiforme and it is Stage 4."

Jack didn't say a word. I could hear Dianne's breathing but not my own. I had stopped breathing.

I said, "How long?"

He said a year, give or take a month or two.

He then added that the tumour was operable, and to give Jack the maximum comfort and time it should be debulked. He had already arranged for Jack to be admitted to Calvary the following Monday for surgery on Tuesday morning.

I remember putting my arm around Jack as we walked out of Andrew's office. Dianne was a couple of feet in front of us and she and I were crying. It was dark and raining outside, and Dianne and I had both driven there separately. She offered to drive me to my car about 500 metres away. I said "no" as it was the only syllable I had left.

I walked to my car, ignoring the rain and feeling nothing. When I finally got there I was soaked, but it didn't matter. I cried like a baby for about ten minutes and felt empty and lost. As a parent you can fix most things with a kiss on the elbow, a Band-Aid or a phone call but I had just been told Jack had 12 months.

I couldn't fix it.

GLIOBLASTOMA MULTIFORME (GBM)

Brain cancer, of which glioblastoma multiforme is one but the most common and the most aggressive, kills more children than any other disease and more people under 40 in Australia than any other cancer (https://engonetcbc2.blob.core. windows.net/assets/uploads/files/Infographic%202017.pdf).

Survival rates for children diagnosed with leukaemia is 87% but for GBM it is 5% and only 20% of people diagnosed with brain cancer will survive for at least five years https://www.curebraincancer.org.au/page/8/facts-stats).

The more I read the more my eyes hurt. How the fuck am I supposed to solve this shit!! There is no way out and everyone dies. Everyone.

THE FIRST OPERATION

Dianne drove Jack to Calvary Hospital for admission on the afternoon of 11 July. I was in the office. Jack could no longer drive, as he needed to be seizure free for at least three months (we were learning a lot about this disease and its implications very quickly).

11 July

Dianne, Jack and I met Andrew Hunn and his assistant in the early evening and we discussed the planned operation (Jack was scheduled first in theatre in the morning) and Jack's ongoing medications. We were told that it was possible that Jack would be on anti-seizure medication for the rest of his life. Wow, I thought, that is not happening!

12 July   When I came back early the next morning, Jack was in his theatre gown and asleep on top of the bed. When I asked him, just after he woke, how he felt, he said he had slept well and was feeling "fine", "not worried" at all. I assumed that this was the truth, but much later he told me that he had been scared about the operation and had slept very little.

The operation went longer than was anticipated. He was meant to go in at 8 and be finished by 11 am. I was anxious that something was not right. Maybe something had gone badly wrong? No, as it turned out, it was the nature of the surgery and the complexity and it took Andrew longer to isolate "all visible" cancer cells that were identified by a fluorescent dye injected into Jack. So, what do you do in the small waiting room outside ICU with a big box of tissues? Well people are coming and going and nobody looks happy and some people are very upset. I cried quietly to myself when I thought no one was looking but there was no shame here, as you only get the chance to sit here when serious shit is going on. It was the waiting room for the imperilled and the damned.

I was scared, really scared, as I was powerless to help my son. I kept Dianne up to date with a few texts and she was on the same emotional rollercoaster. I called her once but typically the sterility of the waiting room and the unspoken fears that were building inside my head, made it difficult to finish the conversation and I hung up. We had already agreed on a rule

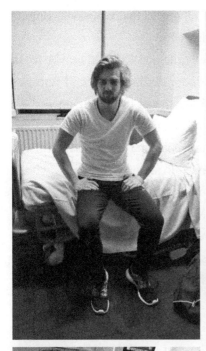

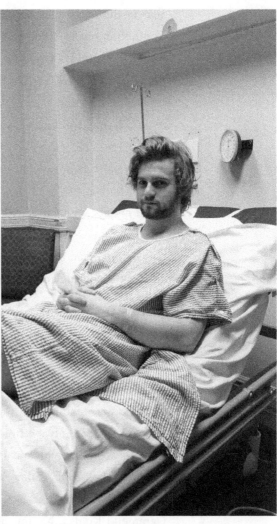

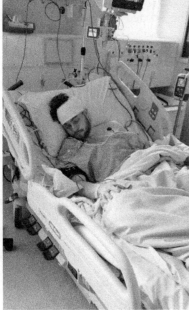

clockwise from top left Arrival,
pre-op and post-op

that in the event that one of us got to that emotional tipping point, then it was OK to just hang up.

I was told it could be a while and I should maybe think about coming back early afternoon. I did and when I returned he was in ICU and asleep. All bandaged up, but he opened his eyes, saw me, smiled and went back to sleep. I cried.

One of the nurses gave me a chair and I sat and stared at him as he went from drowsy awareness to almost comatose. My brain was churning, my eyes were melting, and I felt empty. Dianne came in later with Chris and Matthew. Jack was barely coherent but he smiled a lot and enjoyed the attention. Our conversation was light-hearted and jovial as it would have been before all this shit happened. Hugh couldn't make it and he came in the next day.

13 July Jack was moved to a private ward in the neurology wing the following day.

He was in a lot of pain and needed several doses of morphine over the next couple of days to ease the pain. He was weak, and initially standing and walking were difficult. He slept a lot and naturally was always tired. He ate well, however, although he didn't always finish his meals. We brought in custard tarts each day from the Lenah Valley Bakery (he got that indulgence from me – custard tart with crusty pastry shell). We also brought him Caramello Koalas, his favourites, but he insisted that we take them home to share, as he didn't have an appetite for them.

THE APARTMENT

As the thought that one of our boys would be diagnosed with incurable cancer was equal in consideration to blowing up

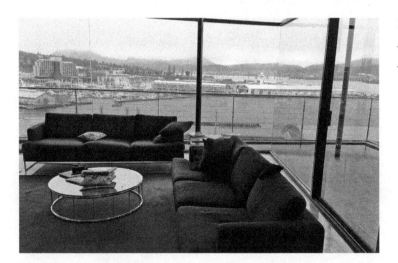

The apartment in Lenna of Hobart, Battery Point

the planet, we had earlier committed to extensive renovation in our home – new kitchen, one new bathroom and laundry makeover. With Jack recovering from major brain surgery and the risk of infection high, it was inconceivable that he could be brought home as it was now a construction site and dust, dirt and workmen were everywhere. The noise would have given even a professional bell-ringer a headache!

So, Jack and I moved into a penthouse at the Lenna for several weeks. On the day Jack was due to be discharged from hospital – 15 July 2016 – we were told he wouldn't be released till the following day – Saturday.

The apartment was a five-minute walk from my office and in the heart of Battery Point so there were plenty of nearby restaurants and bakeries to keep us amused. Dianne stayed at the house in Tranmere with the boys and her brother came down to help her.

I asked Dianne to come in on the Saturday and spend the night, which she did as her brother stayed at the house and

Tasmanian H...

Department of Health and Human Services
ROYAL HOBART HOSPITAL

GPO Box 1061
Hobart, TASMANIA 7001
Ph (03) 6222 8308

Tasmania

RHH
ROYAL HOBART HOSPITAL

Tegretol 200mg	Valproate/Epilim 200mg
Day 1 twice a 1-3 Sat day s. Day 1 = 23/7/16.	1 twice a day 12hrs apart
D4-7 ½ twice a day 26/7 (Tues)	2 twice a day
D 7-9 ½ twice a day 29/7 (Friday)	3 twice a day
D 9 on stop 31/7 (Sunday)	3 twice a day

Dexamethasone
1 whole pill morning
½ pill at dinner

Medication list for dummies (me!)

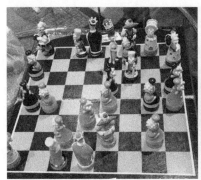 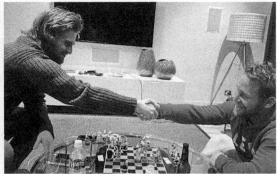

looked after the three boys. We went to dinner and then went to the Grape, 200 metres down the road, for a drink. I ordered a whisky for myself and a gin and tonic for Dianne and we sat and cried our eyes out. "This sucks," she said and we walked back to the apartment.

Jack the victor; Stefan the vanquished

The next day I picked Jack up from Calvary mid-afternoon. I gave him the bedroom with the en suite and I had a separate bedroom.

The first night he came to see me about 1 am complaining of a headache. I gave him some Endone and the pain eased and he went back to sleep. I checked on him several times throughout the night.

This was the time of the Pokémon Go craze and the park below us, Princes Park, was awash with young people searching for Pokémon. In the next couple of days as Jack got stronger he ventured down to the park and indulged in the game.

Stefan flew in from Perth and stayed with us in the apartment. He challenged Jack to chess and regardless of the physical and mental challenges Jack was dealing with, he won each game hands down.

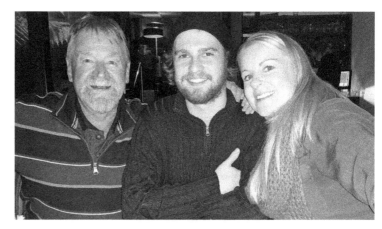

Jack with Casey and Jane Overeem. at Rockwall in Salamanca Place, July 2016

The weather was challenging but Stefan and Jack went out during the day looking for different and more exotic pastries from the various gourmet bakers close to the apartment.

16 July On 16 July, the twins had a football game in Sandy Bay and I went to watch them. It was so cold it snowed, and Chris complained at the end of the game that he couldn't feel his hands. Everyone came back to the apartment for lunch and the boys later went out to chase Pokémon.

Stefan, Jack and I went to a Japanese restaurant in Hampden Road in the evening. It was sleeting (and snowing) while we ate. Jack was animated, as was Stefan as we all forgot about why we were here in the first place and slipped comfortably back into a conversation about the family, friends and the future.

As we sat in the restaurant, I saw a large dog walk slowly past the window. This is not something you see in Hobart and particularly on such a cold night. I thought it was

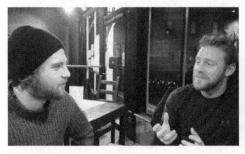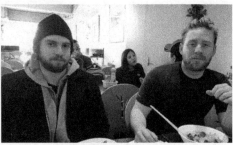

odd and then forgot about it as I re-joined the conversation. When we were leaving the dog wandered back the other way, past the doorway to the restaurant. It was an old dog and it had a white dusting of snow on its fur. It was clearly lost and wouldn't last the night outdoors in this weather. As I turned towards the dog a number of people passed me and looked at its name tag. I don't recall the name but it was an old black Labrador and, typically, very docile. Across the road a small crowd was gathering and everyone was concerned about the dog's wellbeing. The dog however was reluctant to leave the spot where it had stopped, and the conversation turned to, maybe one of the houses close by was its home? Almost as suddenly a door opened, and a man came out and there was obvious recognition between animal and master. He thanked everybody for their concern and mumbled something about someone leaving a gate open and then dog and master disappeared inside the well-lit and obviously very warm home. It was a good ending and I thought at the time that maybe it was a good sign and maybe an omen? But that was wishful thinking.

Jack with Stefan at a Japanese restaurant, left, and at a Vietnamese one for lunch

THE INFORMATION EXPLOSION – FINDING A SOLUTION

Cancer is disease that is "triggered" by a whole lot of things that are no more than theories and conjecture. There are some clear catalysts – bowel, lung and throat cancers, for instance – usually blamed on "lifestyle". Primary brain cancers, on the other hand, have no known triggers. The question was irrelevant for me as knowing the cause did not give the solution, as there wasn't one.

And that was it: full stop.

Well at least for the first 24 hours it was full stop as I had nowhere to go. Snookered by a disease that I hardly knew existed and all the experts telling me just enjoy the next 12 months of his short life. But as I started to read about people who had stared death in the face and lived with GBM (Ben Williams the most notable), clinical trials into new and innovative treatments, promising research, the relationship between diet and cancer and meditation and cancer, my brain exploded.

Jack's tumour was diagnosed as methylated which sounded bad but perversely was good as it meant that "standard" GBM treatment could be followed which was: resection, followed by six weeks of radiation and a course of temozolomide. But it didn't work and, in retrospect, I don't think anything could have saved Jack.

We had to learn a lot quickly. A grand mal seizure is the big one. We now know that Jack's first seizure – 28 May – was a grand mal and even though there were 'instances' when Jack felt an "aura" (he called it) on the periphery of his vision, nothing developed that he couldn't control by sitting down and closing his eyes.

And all the time I was telling him that one day he would be medication free – I was going to figure this out – and there were moments when he honestly believed me.

"I just have to cure the cancer first Jack, and then will sort out the rest. OK?"

"OK."

If I printed all the emails and responses I received and even URLs from web pages I visited, the paper stack would run from the floor to the ceiling and beyond.

BEN WILLIAMS'S 'TRY EVERYTHING AND ANYTHING' DIET (PROBABLY) MATTERS

The book by Ben Williams confirmed my natural prejudice when dealing with medical people–look outside the box and don't believe everything the so-called 'experts' tell you. The documentary Surviving Terminal Cancer, which detailed Ben Williams's story of how he has been able to survive for over 20 years (diagnosed in 1995) with GBM and his book, Surviving "Terminal" Cancer: Clinical Trials, Drug Cocktails, and Other Treatments Your Oncologist Won't Tell You About, gave me hope. My scepticism of medical clinicians and their limitations had been well grounded in my psyche and confirmed by many observations and life experiences. Of note, in 1985 I had attended Camp Eden (health farm) in Currumbin (Queensland) for a six-day course. I went there for all the wrong reasons, but it was life changing as I learnt about the Pritikin diet. In a couple of sentences, Nathan Pritikin was diagnosed with heart disease and told, as most people were in the 1950's, take it easy and go away and die. I recall in the 1970's, a neighbour of my girlfriend at the time, had a heart attack and was immediately retired from work. He was in his early 60's. He was given no dietary or physical exercise advice and told that any exertion could kill him. So, he stayed at home, lived in his dressing gown and watched TV. His only exercise was collecting the morning paper from the front lawn. He ate whatever he liked and whenever he liked. He died shortly thereafter.

Nathan was a fighter, enlightened and curious. He discovered that some primitive cultures that ate little meat and their diet principally consisted of vegetables and fruit, also had very little (or no) history of heart disease. This discovery and research was the premise for his now famous 'Pritikin Diet' – which was low in fat, high in vegetables, fruits, beans, and whole grains, and was combined with moderate exercise. He was treated as a pariah in most medical circles as no one (except a few pioneering souls) accepted the correlation between fat, diet, exercise and heart disease. And even today, people who are candidates for heart disease and diabetes will be given prescriptions rather than advice on diet and exercise. Doctors are great at achieving high marks in exams, healing infections and mending broken bones but completely out of their depth when it comes to dealing (head on) with the lifestyle health epidemic the western world is experiencing today. So, from that pretext, I started with a clean sheet – there is a cure for Jack's brain cancer and someone, somewhere, has the answer and I will find it! Arrogance and self-delusion are cheap commodities.

Ben's philosophical bent was simple: try everything and anything and do not be led by the nose by your oncologists, neurosurgeons and other associated clinicians as they are not risk takers and they follow the book (regardless of the little evidence "the book" saves lives). And in relation to GBM, nothing worked in most cases as most patients were dead within a year – Jack's prognosis – so what was there to lose?

Clinicians have a carefully cultured and prescriptive approach to treatment. And why wouldn't they – with the risk of litigation and reputational damage high for anyone that stepped away from conventional treatments. It was not their job to look beyond the scope of their brief; it was my job. But we all shared one aim and that was to save Jack's life and I could not fault or criticise any one person involved in Jack's care and treatment. I have nothing but the greatest admiration and respect for everyone I met and spoke to and the advice given.

Dianne and I also read a number of 'cancer food' books that argued that certain foods and supplements were cancer fighting. We asked our oncologist about diet and supplements and she was sceptical and said with what he was going through, why compromise and complicate his lifestyle any further? I expected this answer and was respectfully prepared to ignore it. So while Jack was being treated with a cocktail of standard treatments, including daily (and probably permanently) anti-seizure drugs and steroids (dexamethasone), we were adding supplements – turmeric, boswellia, Melatonin and PSK Trammune (to name but a few) – and making major diet changes: green tea, almonds, home-made (raw, unsweetened) muesli, non-fat, plain yoghurt, organic protein shakes (with organic frozen mixed berries, non-fat natural yoghurt and full cream milk), fresh fruit and with garlic and ginger added to most cooked meals. I documented the diet for several weeks and asked Jack to keep track of it, which he (reluctantly) did but eventually he lost complete interest and stopped recording it. And I didn't blame him, between Facebook, watching Arsenal, playing video games and dying of cancer, he was preoccupied.

The more Dianne and I read, the more we corresponded with family and friends, the more we understood, the more hopeful we became about 'non-traditional' therapies and foods as the gateway to Jack's cure. It was empowering and an aphrodisiac. We ran on each other's ether and energy. We started to believe we could find a solution and the answer was somewhere in the maze that constituted the GBM diaspora. Whether anything we did made an ounce of difference we will never know, as we certainly didn't beat the cancer but did we slow it?

Part of my education revealed that many survivors (at least those that were veterans of two years +), had followed Ben's unorthodox approach including volunteering for as many clinical trials as practicable, mixing drugs and supplements (against advice) and maintaining strict dietary regimes, including the ketogenic diet. We looked at the ketogenic ("keto") diet (and revisited it several times) but it was against every principle I had followed for over 30 years (namely it was high in fat) and asymmetric to other dietary advice for fighting cancer. Dianne had a more relaxed attitude to diet than I did but she too baulked at embracing a diet high in fat. Also, and probably more importantly, while Jack was prepared to do anything to beat his cancer, the diet was a bridge too far. Needless to say, it never entered our dietary lexicon (although almost everything else did) until it was too late.

At this point there was becoming a real division of labour between Dianne and I – she did all the heavy lifting with Jack (blood tests, oncology, radiation, neurology, ophthalmologist appointments, filling prescriptions, preparing Jack's meals and dispensing medications) and I spent time in the office as well as trying to find people or clinical trials that maybe could offer a grain of hope.

Jack wasn't allowed to drive anymore following his seizure (one of his greatest frustrations at the time), so Dianne had to drive Jack everywhere. Sometimes we played tag but it was usually Dianne driving (and she did a lot of it back then as the other three boys didn't have a licence and there was shopping to be done, daily school runs, tutoring classes for Matt, football and basketball training and weekend football matches).

I looked at every clinical trial open in the world at that time and contacted the coordinators to test for Jack's eligibility. Also, at that time I was of the view that it didn't matter where the trial was in the world, we would get there if it meant we could save Jack's life. While that was a lofty ideal, the solution was always paramount and the means academic. Well that is the way crusaders' think right, and while there is nothing wrong with that, it was neither practical or realistic.

And I got a lot of feedback and correspondence. I was on a journey. There were many dead ends and "not eligible" responses but others whereby there was the hint of promise and possibilities. Like a rabbit being chased by a fox, I jumped down every rabbit hole and jumped back up again and down another. My correspondence included some of the world's acknowledged brain cancer specialists, including Henry Friedman (Duke) and Patrick Wen (Dana Faber, Harvard). All happy to give their time freely. And what did I discover – no one had any fucking idea how to cure Jack, but information is free. As is talk and dialogue. Just a commodity.

"STANDARD" TREATMENT

After meeting his oncologist, Rosie Harrup, on 1 August 2016, Jack began six weeks of intense radiotherapy, which was to be followed by a course of "chemotherapy" (Temozolomide). During these six weeks he contracted shingles but responded to medication. However, apart from hair loss at the radiation site, Jack generally had few side effects and we were told all blood counts were consistently "great".

After completion of the radiation treatment, the dexamethasone (steroid to reduce brain swelling) was reduced, and then stopped. Jack was pleased as the steroid had several side effects, including a feeling of being always hungry. Subsequently Jack had put on weight and for someone who was always conscious of his weight, and was a fitness junkie, the weight gain was an anathema.

Dianne and I often talked about 'alternative' treatments – high dose Vitamin C, strict (24-hour diet), nutritional and vitamin supplements, meditation, hyperthermia, cannabis oil, etc., and completely walk away from standard established treatments (such as the path we were firmly on). But that requires an intense belief or just bald testosterone to think you have the answer when so many before you had not and the only clinical consensus was that there was no cure. We were never that brave and often now in hindsight, we analyse some of those decisions differently but we were flying blind.

We did however access cannabis oil (at a time its legal status wasn't clear so our channels were clandestine) but we never tested the therapeutic benefits on Jack. It made him wonky and there was just too much going on inside his brain and, combined with the conga line of prescription drugs in his system, we decided it was too experimental to continue.

Life for Jack became very regimented with blood tests every two weeks, radiation every week day for six weeks and meetings with his oncologist and other clinicians. He returned to his studies although his ability to concentrate and comprehend was diminished. He also returned to work and Dianne and I took turns dropping him off and picking him up from the distillery at Cambridge. And there were times when he sensed he was going to have another seizure or his headaches increased, impairing his vision, and he would call Dianne or I (and sometimes both) to come and pick him up.

the next couple of months

Dianne and I were so scared about losing Jack it became difficult to think or talk about anything else. I sent Jack many texts similar to the one I sent on 13 August 2016:

AUGUST

13 August

KEN FLEMING ▸ JACK FLEMING

All good? A world without Jack is not a world I care about. We cannot fail and stand together. But only you, my son, only you can beat this. This is your fight. Win my beautiful son, win because failure is not acceptable.

It also became apparent that he couldn't continue with his studies as he was physically and mentally challenged and although he persevered longer than he should have and I encouraged him longer than I should have, we came to the same realisation. We also agreed that we would "suspend" his studies rather than quit as it was my fervent belief than he would return to his studies in 2017, although that view was not fully accepted by Jack and he was seeing an alternative reality. He did however complete and pass his legal study exams in semester one, year 2, but couldn't sit his Investment Analysis exam as he could no longer comprehend that which he comprehensively and easily understood prior to all this shit going down.

SEPTEMBER

24 September　On 24 September Jack decided to finally put out a post to all his friends on Facebook, most of whom knew a little about Jack's diagnosis:

JACK FLEMING FACEBOOK POST

Its been two and a half months since my world turned upside down and I was diagnosed with glioblastoma multiforme (GBM), a very aggressive brain brain (sic) cancer. There's no real way to determine how or why I developed this, because as with most brain tumours the cause is not known and no apparent clear way to prevent this disease.

I've subsequently undergone a biopsy, brain surgery, have apparently consumed more drugs these past two and a half months than "my dad did in the sixties" (those in the photo barely scratches the surface), and as of tomorrow will have finally completed my final week of the first stage of a six week intense radiotherapy combined with chemotherapy program. I've managed to power through these past six weeks and thankfully with relatively minimal hair loss. In a few weeks I'll have an MRI scan and we will hopefully have some (good) news to report from this and then go from there.

Nothing could have prepared me for everything I've had to endure these past couple of months (and continue to), and I've still got an incredibly long and difficult journey to go. I am not going to sugar-coat it, unfortunately the prognosis for GBM aren't great, but I am not going to let statistics dictate what my

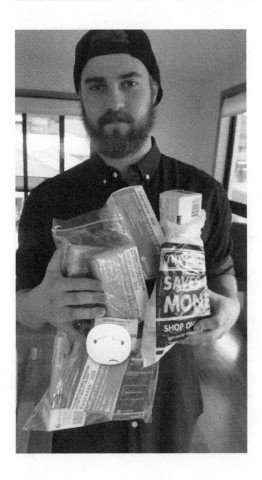

future will be like. This is a fight I have no choice but to stay positive about and I've been taking each day as it comes and will continue fighting with everything I have.

I'm always welcome to answer any questions anyone has regarding this, but know I'm getting through this as well as can be.

Jack

SUPPORT GROUP, HOPE AND DEATHS

I joined a brain cancer support group soon after Jack was diagnosed. There was a lot of information provided by participants, some inspiring and some heart-breaking. Too many deaths.

I relayed Jack's story and received overwhelming support and sympathy and I read many posts, some were helpful, some were heart wrenching and some I responded to if I thought there was a titbit of information worth investigating.

And I cried a lot – so many children and teenagers diagnosed, being treated, suffering and succumbing. Some were long posts and some were short – asking to be taken off the email contact list as the person they were writing about was no longer alive. What the fuck was I dealing with? So much tragedy and I, we, knew nothing.

But I think my story of Jack inspired others as well, at least in the beginning and when I asked to be taken off the list in April, given that I knew his time was short, I received many heart-warming messages.

In the beginning there was surety in numbers and there was always that belief we would find the Holy Grail and I could share the joy. But in the end, like so many other families, I shared the pain.

OCTOBER

3 October

Second

grand mal

seizure

On 3 October 2016 he had his second, grand mal, seizure. This is not something I would recommend watching for the faint-hearted, particularly when it is your child. He had come home from the Lark Distillery, and said he was feeling a "little funny". He said, "This is not good," and started to shake violently. He was on a bar stool and as I grabbed him he collapsed. Matthew grabbed his left side and we lowered him to the floor and put a pillow under his head.

We called the ambulance but, after speaking to the para-medics, we decided to watch him at home as he recovered reasonably quickly and the seizure lasted just a few minutes.

The following day he woke with a mild headache, which started to build in intensity. After he vomited, and the Panadol didn't work, we again called an ambulance and took him to hospital, where they gave him some morphine to reduce the pain. Worried his tumour had returned, Jack requested a follow up MRI but it showed no sign of a tumour.

It was conjectured by his oncologist that the rapid re-duction of the dexamethasone dose probably caused the seizure, so Jack was returned to dexamethasone with the dosage to be reduced over time.

When Jack was advised by the UTAS that he had failed "Investment Analysis" (as he couldn't sit the exam) he got angry, as he knew without his diagnosis and treatment he would have been awarded a High Distinction (HD). I wrote to the university and made a compelling case for reconsideration based on his internal marks and my appeal fell on sympathetic ears with the informal comment that this was ridiculous as he was a "star" student and they agreed he would have passed the exam without effort. I sent Jack the following text:

K: You have been awarded a HD in Investment Analysis! **14 October** Professor of Economics and Finance at the School of Business, Mardi Dungey, just rang me to congratulate you. Congratulations Jack. Well deserved. Dad.

On 18 October he began a six-month course of temozolomide. **18 October** Five days on and 25 days off. He had few noticeable side effects;

his blood counts were good and he managed to return to full-time work, as he was no longer studying

NOVEMBER

15 November

Second month (15 November) temozolomide dose was increased and again with few affects, mainly tiredness. Blood work remained good, but headaches returned, and Endone was often needed.

DECEMBER

16 December

Friday 16 December, Jack came home early (2 pm) from work with a headache, which paracetamol then Endone did not seem to help. At 1.30 am, Dianne drove Jack to hospital as he was now vomiting, unable to keep water down, becoming dehydrated, and in severe pain.

Headaches had become a new vernacular for us and Jack was rarely free of head pain. The most potent of his prescription medications for headaches was Endone (which included a mild dose of morphine) and while we used it frequently, Jack often complained that he didn't like the "spaced out" feeling he got after taking it and wasn't convinced it made any difference. We put the headaches down to swelling which was associated with his earlier surgery and the belief (naïve as it turned out) that the temozolomide was doing its job and killing the cancer cells and thus contributing to the swelling and consequent headaches. We thus thought he was having a negative reaction to the temozolomide and nothing else and maybe the dexamethasone dose was too low.

You see, we had no idea but plenty of theories. All of which may have been logical but this time we were completely out of our depth and were about to get a second (and equally) sobering lesson on this evilness of this disease.

In hospital, the medical staff managed to get his headache down and he settled only after high dose IV morphine was administered. He finally got some sleep. Dianne left around 9 am on Saturday and came home and I arrived at the hospital just after she left. It was decided to send Jack for a CT scan.

17 December

The scan led to a request for an MRI. I didn't think much about it at the time and thought it was just standard medical procedure given the nature of Jack's illness. Jack came back to the ward and we were told to wait for the results. Within an hour we were told that Andrew Hunn was doing his "normal hospital rounds" and was coming down to see Jack. We were asked to wait.

I assumed that this was a courtesy call. Jack said he was worried as there would be no reason for Andrew to see him unless the news was bad. I said, "That's bullshit." I looked forward to proving him wrong. However, he was convinced the news was not good and he was visibly nervous. So we waited; neither of us saying much but there was a lot going on in our collective heads that was saying a lot.

When Andrew arrived, he got straight to the point: the MRI showed some possible tumour regrowth. But, he emphasised, in this early time period post radiation it can be difficult to tell if changes represent tumour regrowth or a phenomenon of pseudoprogression (which is essentially a treatment inflammatory effect). The latter was the view that his oncologist held (although Andrew was more sceptical and thought it was tumour regrowth). He scheduled Jack for a biopsy and, if the biopsy confirmed tumour regrowth,

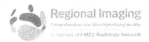

Regional Imaging
Comprehensive care. Uncompromising quality.
A member of I-MED Radiology Network

Medical Imaging Report

Dr Erica Kreismann
A & E DEPT. CALVARY HOSPITAL
49 AUGUSTA ROAD
LENAH VALLEY TAS 7008

Calvary Hospital

RE: Mr Jack Fleming   DOB: 25/11/1996   Age: 20 Years

Visit Number: 9457573
MRN: HC227453

Date of Examination: 17/12/2016

Referred By: Dr Erica Kreismann
Report Date: 17/12/2016

MRI BRAIN

CLINICAL NOTES
Headache and vomiting for 4 days. GBM diagnosed June 2016, currently on chemo.

TECHNIQUE
Pre and post contrast MRI brain including diffusion and susceptibility imaging.

COMPARISON STUDY
CT brain today, MRI brain 14/10/16 and prior.

FINDINGS
The previous MRI study from October 2016 demonstrated mild vasogenic oedema within the left parietal occipital lobe. This has shown significant increase compared to the previous study. Effacement of the posterior horn of the left lateral ventricle, otherwise the ventricles are not dilated. New mild midline shift towards the right of 5mm. Please see the saved image.

In the region of the debulking procedure, there is extensive patchy new high signal change on T2 and FLAIR weighted imaging anteromedially, suggestive of extensive recurrent tumour. This area shows peripheral extensive enhancement post administration of Gadolinium. Compared to the pre operative study, the degree of enhancement has shown marked progression. Mildly restricted diffusion in this area. SWI artefact in the region of previous debulking, but not in the new enhancing tumour.

In the right frontal lobe white matter, there is no enhancing lesion, however, there is mild oedema, and extensive white matter hyperintensity throughout the left centrum semiovale. This is stable from previous, as are the multiple small cystic areas throughout the white matter of the left cerebral hemisphere.

No cerebellopontine angle mass. The 3rd and 4th ventricles are normal. Major intracranial flow voids are preserved.

Soft tissue thickening throughout the right maxillary sinus is new consistent with sinusitis.

Page: 1 (cont...)

Ken.
Jacks Dad — please phone
when ready

Regional Imaging Pty Ltd

Head Office
PO Box 5076 Brandon Park VIC 3150
T: 03 9587 5100 F: 03 8587 5189
E: enquiries@regionalimaging.com.au
regionalimaging.com.au

A member of I-MED Radiology Network
i-med.com.au

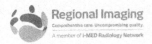

Regional Imaging
Comprehensive care. Uncompromising quality.
A member of I-MED Radiology Network

Medical Imaging Report

Dr Mark Baldock
A & E DEPT. CALVARY HOSPITAL
49 AUGUSTA ROAD
LENAH VALLEY TAS 7008

Calvary Hospital

RE: Mr Jack Fleming DOB: 25/11/1996 Age: 20 Years

Visit Number: 9457316
MRN: HC227453

Referred By: Dr Mark Baldock
Date of Examination: 17/12/2016   Report Date: 17/12/2016

CT BRAIN - JACK FLEMING

CLINICAL DATA
GBM debulked 12/7/2016. MRI 14/10/2016 baseline. Increasing headaches. ? Aetiology. ? Cerebral oedema.

FINDINGS
Comparison was made with the previous CT brain dated 4/10/2016 and MRI brain dated 14/10/2016.
Since the previous studies, extensive vasogenic type cerebral oedema has developed in the left frontoparietal lobe, with extension into the occipital lobe. There is compression of the adjacent left lateral ventricle and there is mild midline shift to the right by 4mm.
Previous overlying left parietal craniotomy is noted.
Multiple small cystic areas in the right frontoparietal lobe, with hypodense changes in the surrounding cerebral white matter are unchanged compared to previously.

CONCLUSION
Extensive vasogenic type cerebral oedema has developed in the left frontoparietal lobe, with extension into the occipital lobe, implies recurrent tumour. Tumour mass not seen, and therefore repeat CT brain post-contrast or ideally MRI brain is recommended to further evaluate. Significant mass effect with compression of the left lateral ventricle and midline shift to the right by 4mm.
Results telephoned at 8.55am.

Thank you for referring this patient.

Mei Pang

CC: Rhh Oncology Unit Rhh Oncology Unit, Dr Rosemary Harrup, Dr Alison Kinnane

Regional Imaging Pty Ltd
ABN 81 095 630 792
Head Office
PO Box 5038, Brandon Park VIC 3150
T: 03 8587 5380 F: 03 8587 5189
E: enquiries@regionalimaging.com.au
regionalimaging.com.au

A member of I-MED Radiology Network
i-med.com.au

immediate surgery on 20 December. The pathology would be undertaken at the beginning of the surgery and, if the diagnosis was confirmed as Andrew expected, surgery to "debulk" the tumour would immediately follow.

THE SECOND OPERATION

20 December I again expected the operation (if necessary) to be around three hours but again, it went on longer. I went to the hospital at 11 and was told that Jack was not out yet and Andrew would call me. I had some lunch and Andrew called and said it was tumour regrowth and he had removed as much of the tumour as was visible. He had arranged with the medical staff to give me access to the Recovery Unit where Jack was being treated before he was moved to the ICU (Intensive Care Unit).

I drove back to the hospital and waited outside the Recovery Unit and a medical person ushered me into the Unit to see Jack. He was barely conscious but managed a smile when he saw me and then closed his eyes and dosed. He had tubes and bandages everywhere and I cried. One of the nurses saw me and came over to comfort me and she started crying. A second nurse also came over and put her arms around us both. After a couple of minutes, I kissed him on the forehead and left. I returned an hour later to see him again in ICU.

I sent a text to Andrew and asked if it was possible to see him later that day to discuss the operation and what he found during surgery. He agreed to see me at 5 pm in his consulting rooms. The discussion was frightening, confronting and

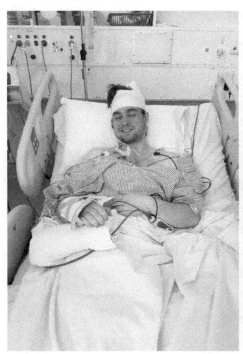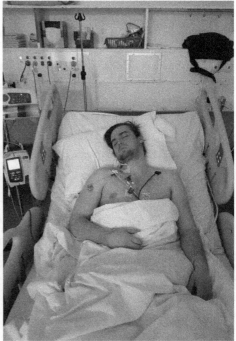

left me gutted, again. He said the tumour was in same place although deeper and "five" times larger than the original tumour. He advised that he had managed to remove all visible signs of the tumour but said given the size and timing, he would be lucky to survive a further six months as the tumour was "very aggressive".

I cried and he came around to my side of the desk and comforted me. He told me to stay in the waiting room as long as I wanted and said he was very very sorry, but "it is what it is". That expression became part of the unavoidable (and growing) vernacular that defined our horrible journey with this disease.

CHRISTMAS EVE 2016
and the days that followed

24 December   Andrew rang me in the morning of 24 December and said he was comfortable releasing Jack from hospital in the afternoon. Thought he was well enough to spend Christmas at home. I recall the phone call vividly as I was hanging clothes out on the washing line when the phone rang in my pocket. We did not expect Jack to be released till after Christmas so this was a GREAT Christmas present.

However, I was now convinced that this would be his last Christmas and the last conversation with Andrew weighed on me heavily as the message was clear and I was the one that would have to tell Jack. Jack, on the other hand, was in good spirits and as I later found out, he was of the view that the worst was behind him. He was devastated when I finally found the courage to discuss this with him and, while never a person who showed deep emotion, Jack was shaken.

That conversation came after the older boys had left Hobart and returned home, as I wanted Jack to enjoy the time he had left and he would be denied nothing. They typically took control of Jack's life while they were down, taking him everywhere and played games with him most days. I told them privately what Andrew had told me, that the prognosis was poor and this would be his last Christmas although I also tempered these conversations with comments about new drugs, trials, and stories of survival. And Jack was not dead and didn't look like dying; it was easy for them (and myself sometimes) to believe my own bullshit.

After his release, he experienced (predictably) ongoing headaches, although generally he was more settled and there was less discomfort than the period directly following his first surgery.

He was due to commence his fourth dose of temozolomide on 10 January, but this was replaced with lomustine, which he started on 4 January 2017. The decision to switch from temozolomide to lomustine was recommended by his oncologist and coincidentally confirmed later by the pathology results provided by Manuel Graeber and Michael Buckland who graciously reviewed Jack's original pathology results and diagnosis. They were my January project and it opened up another rabbit hole for me, which I readily jumped down – always prepared to chase everything and anyone who I sensed offered a ray of hope (no matter how obtuse and thin that hope was).

26 December

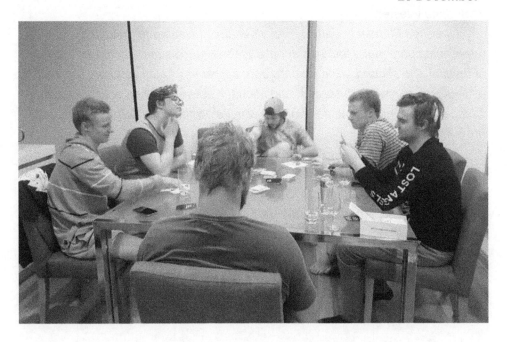

MANUEL AND MICHAEL: PAEDRIATIC GBM

Probably the most significant and rewarding communication was with Professor Manuel Graeber (Barnet-Cropper Chair of Brain Tumor Research, Brain and Mind Centre, University of Sydney). My contact with him came via a circuitous route but he took the view that he was interested in Jack's case as he felt his tumour should not be so aggressive in "someone so young". He felt there was a possibility (albeit slim) of a misdiagnosis. I was sceptical but hopeful that maybe, just maybe, he was right! He works closely with Dr Michael Buckland (Head of the Department of Neuropathology at Royal Prince Alfred Hospital, Head of the Molecular Neuropathology Program at the Brain & Mind Research Institute). Michael agreed with Manuel to test the tumour and thereby validate (or not) the original diagnosis. Michael was on leave but agreed on his return in early January, that Jack's tumour would be immediately tested.

I visited Manuel in early January because I wanted to make this relationship personal. I told him about Jack's diagnosis and gave him copies of the first and second MRIs (prior to both surgeries). I also included a photo of Jack as I wanted both Manuel and Michael, as well as their colleagues, to associate the tumour (and its analysis) with its owner. Jack was a person and not a tissue sample.

The report was dated 9 January 2017 and confirmed the original diagnosis – glioblastoma multiforme grade 4. Contained in the report, however, was this observation: "Given the patient's age at diagnosis, this tumour is best classified as an AYA (adolescents and young adults, 15-39) glioblastoma, IDH-wildtype, WHO (2016) grade IV". Otherwise referred to as "Paediatric GBM". What I didn't know then, and the significance of the report finding was lost on me at the time, was that paediatric GBM's are typically more aggressive and do not normally respond to temozolomide. This was also the view that Jack's oncologists were forming as Jack had not responded to his, up until this point, traditional GBM treatment of: surgery, radiation and temozolomide.

Jack's oncologist passed Jack onto her new colleague, John Heath, who had experience with paediatric GBM in Melbourne. Following Jack's second operation in December, Rosie had recommended that we abandon temozolomide and replace it with lomustine – a more potent drug and one that had been around for some time and had shown some success against GBM.

And while we thought the observation regarding the higher aggression of GBM tumours in young people was salient, in hindsight, we were just shuffling deck chairs on the Titanic because nothing, I repeat, nothing, was going to stop this ship from going down. But in hindsight we are all smarter and at that time, at that point in Jack's short history, we all felt this was a watershed moment.

calendar 2017

4 January   HE STARTED LOMUSTINE ON 4 JANUARY 2017.

During January, he started walking every day and drinking our "crazy carrot-based" drinks but did not complain. We also helped him prepare his Will (everything goes to his five brothers) and had many frank discussions to which his usual retort was "in other words, I am fucked".

I recall this was a difficult subject to broach for obvious reasons and even more emotionally treacherous to execute. There are no levels of pain here and everything was a 10, however traversing the delicate discussions with your 21-year-old son on the necessity to write a Will, and then helping him prepare it, was a 10+. I do remember one lighter moment when he said he was leaving everything to his brothers and he then looked at me with that cheeky grin of his and said "you've got too much so you don't need it"! Correct I smiled back and thought there is only one thing I want from you Jack and you can't give it to me.

Jack is good. No side effects from first dose of lomustine last night (expect some hair loss though?). Have re-started diet restrictions and added health drink (Aloe Vera, celery, ginger, apple and orange). Jack walking every day, losing weight and feeling better. Tumour tests to be completed next week in Sydney (don't expect news to be good); have referrals to several Melbourne institutions and have been in touch with Head of Dana Faber (Harvard) re Jack and "options".

11 January

We might be able to add weeks or months but doubt there is anything out there at present that will get him to his 21st and another Christmas. But won't stop trying until he says "enough".

Jack went out tonight with friends and was in good spirits.

13 January

Royal Children's Hospital (RCH) in Melbourne very keen to get into Jack's case. Waiting on pathological review to be completed by Sydney University. Not sure where this leads but response from RCH was quite pointed in the level of testing required and the Sydney academics have been in touch with RCH to accommodate. The response from RCH was also a little more upbeat than I had envisaged but a lot hinges on the DNA mapping of the tumour. I am out of my depth but Professor Manuel Graeber seems to have taken this on at a personal level, which is humbling. Even refused a bottle of fine Lark whisky as "will not accept any financial benefit".

email MICHAEL BUCKLAND ▸ KF

17 January

Dear Ken

I have reviewed this case with Manuel, including some additional stains and molecular tests.

We both agree with the Hobart pathologists – this is a Glioblastoma, WHO grade 4.

I have asked for a couple of the tests to be repeated due to some technical issues with the stains, so the final report won't be completed until tomorrow. We shall send it through to you and the relevant doctors tomorrow.

Kind regards Michael

Michael Buckland MBBS PhD FRCPA

21 January Spoke to Dr Patrick Wen from Harvard (Dana Faber) this morning. Reinforced our view that here is as good as anywhere for treatment and there is a huge emotional and financial cost attached to going overseas. Said best people to talk to in Australia are Mark Rosenthal and Mustafa Khasraw – both of whom we are already in touch with.

He also talked about off-label immunotherapy drugs that we will investigate.

The introduction to Dr Wen came from Manuel who knew him personally and we were humbled that he would call us to discuss Jack's case. We were also comforted by the fact that there was nothing in the GBM universe that we couldn't access locally and we were not prejudicing Jack's health by keeping him in Australia.

Also, now have a referral to Dr Zeigler at Sydney Children's Hospital at Randwick. He is back on Monday.

24 January **email MICHAEL BUCKLAND ▸ KF**

Dear Ken

I am glad that you may have found a trial for Jack. You are in good hands with David Ziegler.

We are about to trial a new deep sequencing panel looking at identifying druggable mutations in solid tumours. It is designed mainly for tumours like breast, colon and lung cancer, but it does have some glioblastoma relevant targets. It is called Oncomine comprehensive cancer panel from Thermo Fisher.

Thermo have offered to run one sample for us free of charge so we can evaluate the panels usefulness for brain tumours. Would you consent for us to send Jack's tumour to them for this evaluation?

As this is really a first look at this new technology I doubt that we will uncover anything particularly useful for Jack's treatment, so please don't get your hopes up. It may not even work. If you would prefer us not to use Jack's tumour that is fine too as we have research material that we can send in his place. If you consent to using Jack's tumour then we will share the report with Dr Ziegler and Dr Hansford and anyone else that you would like us to. It will be a 'research only' report as the assay is not yet clinically validated.

Kind regards

Michael

MICHAEL BUCKLAND MBBS PhD FRCPA FFSc (RCPA

email DAVID ZIEGLER, Sydney Children's Hospital ▸ KF   **25 January**

Thanks for your emails and I'm very sorry to hear about Jack's diagnosis and progress.

Unfortunately, our hospital does not allow us to accept patients above the age of 16 years. We often try and argue the case and have in the past been able to get patients seen here up to 18 years of age, but they won't take older patients than that.

The agent we are testing in the trial has already been tested in the adult population, so one thing we could consider is approaching the company to see if they would be prepared to supply the drug on a compassionate basis for a young adult patient. They have treated patients in Melbourne before, so that may be possible, or the other option would be to find an adult hospital in Sydney that would be prepared to use this novel agent.

Would you be happy for me to forward Jack's information to the drug company?

Many thanks

David Ziegler

I responded with an emphatic "yes".

27 January Through a mutual friend, I contacted Dr Kathy Tucker (Prince of Wales Hospital, NSW) who apprised me of the "MoST" program at The Garvan Institute of Medical Research. Kathy forwarded me the following response from Garvan:

forwarded email
The Garvan Institute of Medical Research ▸
DR KATHY TUCKER, Prince of Wales Hospital
It all depends on how well he is, Kathy. We're trying not to raise undue expectations for patients and their families, especially when they have to travel a long way. The major issue in this case will be performance status: he'd need to be 0-2 (i.e., self-caring), and actually 0-1 for the immunotherapy study. This is difficult for family to estimate accurately, so it's best we liaise with his oncologist.

Could you perhaps ask his Dad to mention the study and contact details (MoST@garvan.org.au) to his oncologist, and we can determine his eligibility and the utility therefore of coming up to visit?

Hope this helps

Kathy

30 January

Had a meeting with Jack's oncologist today. She is following up on all my leads and was complimentary of the work undertaken in Sydney by Manuel and Michael as it showed that Jack's tumour has some important "receptors" which can be targeted. This information would not normally be available unless forensic testing had been undertaken and which, incidentally, Manuel and Michael had completed.

Jack agreed to return on Friday to meet the new head of Oncology at the Royal, a "paediatric oncologist" specialising in GBMs. He is ex-Royal Children's Hospital in Melbourne so could be fortuitous.

email DR GEORGE L ▸ KF　　　　　　　　　　　　**31 January**

Subject: RE: Jack Fleming, diagnosed with GBM #4

Dear Ken,

Did you have any news from the RCH or Dr L?

If nothing available, we might be able to look more into that EGFR positive expression.

There is an investigational drug ABT414 that we might be able to access via compassionate scheme.

But I would give priority to a clinical trial if one available and Jack eligible.

We could still chase this later if trial option doesn't work and nothing else available.

Kind regards

George L

FEBRUARY

3 February Found this note when I got up as Jack not in the house:

Feel really good but can't sleep past 3.45 despite taking pill.
Will take my phone.
It's now 7 am.

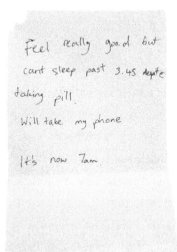

7 February Late last year we set up a WhatsApp message group for my family.

WhatsApp POST

Just to bring you all up-to-date on where we are at with Jack:

1   Jack's oncologist was following up with Garvan;

2   David Ziegler has referred Jack to the "drug" company and since advised that the drug company was contacting "your doctor in Hobart" as "have a trial opening in Melbourne which they thought he might be eligible for". He advised me of this on 6 February;

3   Victoria (Jack's consulting nurse) had followed up with Epworth in Melbourne (Dr Jason L who was referred to me by Dr George L [Medical Oncology Research Fellow

Olivia Newton-John Cancer & Wellness Centre] and had passed that information onto Rosie);

4   Dr George L had also advised me that he might be able to access drugs on "compassionate grounds" if I had no luck elsewhere. I advised Victoria of this on 6 February;

5   Dr Michael Buckland (Sydney Uni) is arranging for additional forensic testing of Jack's tumour.

Jack well considering but platelets are very low and thus he is vulnerable to viruses/bugs, etc. He is off the steroids and sleeping soundly through the night (usually he would wake around 2 am and struggle to get back to sleep). He is eating well and exercising most days. His general demeanour however is dour, moody and generally uncommunicative. There is a bit of the old Jack there (he was always more serious and very quiet) but can blame a lot of the rest on the cocktail of drugs he is on. He is also cutting back on his seizure medication (all of which is helping him feel a little better).

I can push his oncologist to accelerate these contacts, but this is the public health system. That said, she is also looking at accessing other drugs on "compassionate grounds" to assist Jack and we have no reason to believe the drug is not working. I think his next MRI is next week and that may (I fear) show some progression of the tumour.

From the perspective of Dianne and I, we want to see what the Garvan Institute has to offer and hopefully (just maybe?) they can deal with all his medications, processing and vision issues in one holistic process.

The "drug" referred to above is lomustine (chemotherapy). His next dose is expected to be on 22/23 February. He had a blood test on Monday (yesterday) and they want another on Wednesday (tomorrow) as there is real concern re his platelets.

11:35 am Yes talking to Jack can be prickly. Gotta pick your moments. Garvan does sound interesting though. But pushing the public health system to respond is like pulling teeth. That said, I know I have bombarded Hobart Oncology with requests and referrals and they have been pretty good. However, I just have five months left to get it right and that does make this parent a little antsy.

5.31 pm These are my notes (just keeping everyone in the loop):

1   The Nivolumab is an option that can be administered locally but it has been primarily used for other cancers and has had mixed success with brain tumours. However, she said that there was a cost: $3,500 per dose and it needs to be taken every three weeks. There is a "30% compassionate" discount though. Oncologist will investigate if there is any additional financial assistance she can arrange;

2   ABT414 is a "targeted agent" (Stage 3 trial phase although no results have been published) and that has been administered (and used) here is Tasmania in conjunction with lomustine. She is very familiar with the drug and its side effects (including drying of the eyes). It can be administered here and she will pursue. She also added that the analysis of Jack's tumour in Sydney has identified a number of receptors that can be targeted and that is "good";

3   She has spoken to Epworth (Melbourne) and advised that there are no current clinical trials that would be applicable to Jack. There are a number of Phase 1 trials at Epworth for brain cancer and other cancers but not recommended as Phase 1 is measuring "toxicity" and not "efficacy";

4   She was going to follow up email from George L at Austin to see what he has available;

5   She is also going to follow up the Garvan Institute to see also what treatments are available (as would appear that Jack might be eligible);

6   She asked that I get in touch with David Ziegler and she gave me her mobile # (– – –) so that she can follow up his email re the drug company that was "going to contact her re clinical trials about to start in Melbourne". I have since emailed David;

7   Finally, I said that I would confirm with Michael Buckland that there is sufficient tumour left to undertake additional analysis in the event that Jack was a candidate for assistance at Garvan or a clinical trial. I phoned Grace (Heng) Wei (who is assisting Michael on further analysis of Jack's tumour) on 7 February and she said that she would check with Michael and advise.

Jack had his first MRI post-surgery yesterday. ALL CLEAR!!!!!!!!!   **17 February**

Oncologist (as we all did) expected regrowth so was happily slain by result. No work as yet. Agreement is if he gets two clean slates it is back to Uni.   **18 February**

Also planning to take him to Sydney in March. Hope to go to Mum's on Monday 20 March and catch up with you all? Everything depends on his health and well enough to fly. Barring a disaster however I should be there then at least. Does that work with everybody?

19 February Back in hospital. At friend's house last night and it was dark; he ran into a wall playing football. Head banged up pretty badly (can't see from this [left] photo) and broke a finger. Unf**kingbelievable! And lost his phone. Di spent good part of evening in hospital and back there now. Being released in next 20 minutes. He was taken there in an ambulance.

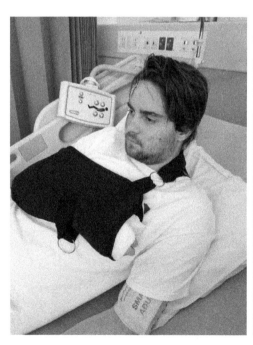
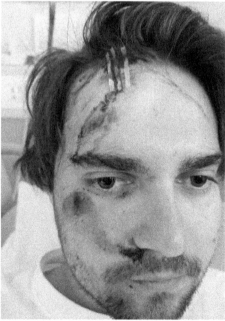

20 February

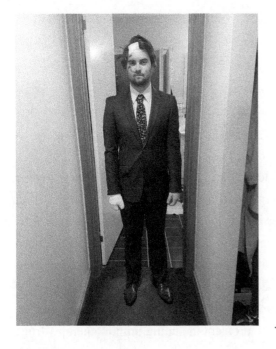

Nick Burk's wedding (Jack a mess but nothing would have stopped him from going!):

On 25 February, he received his second lomustine dose. Again, well-tolerated by Jack, although bloods were showing temporary reduced platelets and care taken. Minimal hair loss, mild rash, no nausea, increased tiredness but sleeping well.

25 February

WhatsApp POST

Brief update. Jack all good; Di had a birthday on 8 March (happy birthday Lily) and I had my annual blood test (results improved significantly across the board). On the blood test, Dr refusing to see me and sent out some big ticks on the results sheets. Usual story. Given stress of Jack and constricted activity post knee op, thought health would be worse. But nup, I think there is a contra going on between Jack and I: the sicker he gets the healthier I get. Really sucks.

MARCH

10 March

Jack has no adverse symptoms either from the chemo or associated with cancer but I am not going to be encouraged given we were poleaxed pre-Christmas.

Looking forward to a whisky or several tonight as liver count the best in 15 years. Dianne reckons that is so unfair and she is right!!

17 March   A number of paths led to the Garvan Institute in Sydney re some innovative treatments for rare cancers. I started the conversation with Kathy Tucker and as a coincidence had dinner in Hobart in February with an ex-Director of the Garvan. He introduced me to his contacts at Garvan and I received this response from Dominique H. I cried when I received it as my understanding of the MoST program was that anything and everything would be thrown at solving the problem including immunotherapy drugs that couldn't be assessed outside of a current clinical trial. The only code, from my understanding, was solve the problem no matter what it takes and when you have only months left we had nothing to lose and everything to gain.

forwarded email DOMNIQUE H ▸ KF

Subject: Re: jack fleming

Please find attached an information sheet on the MoST program for Jack Fleming's oncologist. It outlines the process for referrals and the documentation we require for enrolment. The referral letter and documents can be sent to most@ garvan.org.au or faxed to ––.

Once we receive the referral we will contact Mr Fleming to schedule an appointment at the Kinghorn Cancer Centre.

Also attached is the Participant Information and Consent Form for more information on what participation in the molecular screening component of the MoST program involves.

Please let me know if you would like further information.

Kind regards,

Dominique

WhatsApp POST   **19 March**

Jack doing more maths and joking with Hugh. Just came down to joke with me. Could almost pretend life is normal …?   1.54 pm

Don't mention Garvan with Jack when we are up there pls. Di and I have found he just wants to be led and gets very confused and frustrated when we talk about different treatment options.   1.56 pm

But Garvan is my killer punch. All the documents have been sent to me so starting to get that going.   1.57 pm

One small thing about Jack that he doesn't like me mentioning in front of him is his hearing problem. He is good if you face him, but he generally misses a lot. I tend to speak a little louder when he is around. Sometimes his answers don't fit the question so don't worry about repeating it.

He is looking forward to it, especially his favourite food which I will get him tomorrow: wonton noodle soup with BBQ pork!

Jack has a headache all day. That is a very very bad sign. He is worried; parents really f..ked up. Don't respond to this post pls. We know what this means. If he has a headache-free day tomorrow I will tell you. He knows, he knows, and he is scared.   **24 March**

25 March
10.02 am

No headache! Feeling good; had a good night's sleep. Hallelujah!

11.06 am

Jack just came down to talk to me. He was not being honest when I spoke to him earlier. Had a headache all morning and sudden loss of vision. These are the classic signs of the tumour growing again.

We had a frank discussion and I didn't sugar-coat what this means. He is upset but it is what it is.

7.46 pm

We have had some confronting conversations. He is depressed.

I am over bullshit. I have lied to him and myself because it was easy. Pretend it will end well. Not anymore. He deserves, needs and wants my honesty. It hurts, it hurts but he is my son and I am over the bullshit.

Adrian and Stefan down:

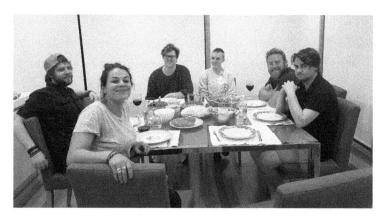

Missing the twins. Cara is Matt's girlfriend and Ingrid "Frenchie" is Adrian's squeeze

26 March

Did any of you get any sleep??

I did. Whisky helped. Di not sure but she is in a good mood at the moment as Jack up and in great spirits. Head is better and he has been wrestling with Hugh. Big smile on his face.

I wouldn't read too much into it though as we are all pretty
certain tumour back. Play it day-by-day.

> *Ok ... thanks ... we are all anxiously waiting ...*   11.06 am
> *everything crossed.*

Moving on Garvan tomorrow. No time to waste. MRI ASAP   11.11 am
and see where it sits. If operable then consider that first to
remove pressure on the brain and then get Garvan moving.
Not sure when he can fly after operation but the op, if feasible,
will give us another 3 months.

Had lunch on Tuesday with a couple of people out at Manly.   11.36 am
Talked about Jack. One of the guys said he went to a funeral
the previous week of a 12-year-old girl who died of GBM.
She was diagnosed in June, like Jack so only got 10 months.
Family devastated. Also, in the GBM support group I am in,
one guy asked to be taken off the mailing list as his daughter,
23, had just died. She also only got 10 months, diagnosed in
June, same as Jack.

Sucks. Just sucks.

MRI organised for 2.45 today. Neurosurgeon will call me   **27 March**
this evening with results. Dianne working with oncologist to
fast track Garvan if possible. Jack however a lot better and
headache is about 1 out of 10 and sometimes not there at all.
He was playing board games with his two older brothers and
Ingrid till about 3 am and just woke up.

MRI done, now wait for results. Garvan has all of Jack's   4.11 pm
paperwork. Oncologist was coincidentally at Garvan last week
and everyone knows Jack Fleming.

6.32 pm   Dodged a bullet. No sign of tumour, no change since last MRI. Cavity has "shrunk" which means brain matter regrowth. Have oncology meeting Friday.

Jack over the moon. Can't get the smile off his face.

However, speaking to Andrew Hunn the next day, he commented:

Text ANDREW HUNN ▸ KF

Further to our conversation last evening, I have reviewed Jack's films with radiology. There is little change between the scan in February and yesterday's scan, but on both there is an area behind the resection cavity that is most likely tumour. It has not changed appreciably between the two scans, which may mean that the lomustine is holding it at this stage.

30 March   Hope grows where despair once was only present.

I contacted the university and said Jack is thinking of resuming his studies. This is the response I got from Mardi:

email MARDI ▸ KF

Sent: Thursday, March 30, 2017 5:07 pm

To: Ken Fleming

Cc: Nagaratnam

Subject: Hi Ken

We are so pleased to hear from you – Sree must have told you that we had only been talking about Jack yesterday. I am sorry I wasn't in the office today to talk with you.

I would be more than delighted to talk with Jack at any time he feels ready and figure out something that he might like to do. I am more than happy to talk with him about perhaps doing a course of study with me or Sree or perhaps doing a project together.

I am so glad that things are going better than expected at this stage – we have been thinking of you and worrying for you.

Jack might like to come and be part of our 'economics club' events for example when we have them – I think there will be one next Friday afternoon, but we can let you know.

SO glad to hear from you and Jack.

Mardi*
Professor of Economics and Finance University of Tasmania

WhatsApp POST

APRIL

1 April

Forgot to mention but view is that recurrence of headaches is possibly due to cavity shrinkage which ironically is a good thing.

Jack also said to us as we left the oncologist that there could come a time when he will choose quality of life over quantity. He said there is only so much of this he can, and is, prepared to take and there could come a day when he says no more.

We said we understand and would support any decision, no matter how painful, he makes.

Jack played a game today that he bought in November and struggled with. His brain functions are returning. He found it too difficult previously and ignored it. Today was a watershed moment. Light bulbs going off everywhere inside his head as his brain rebuilds. He was so chuffed.

---

*   Professor Mardi Dungey died on 12 January 2019 following a short illness. She's fondly remembered by this family.

3 April   All jokes aside he is in as a good a shape as anytime in the last 9 months. Joking, chasing the twins, arguing with Matt. Close my eyes and we are almost back, pre-June last year. Also did a major eye test today as a precursor to driving again. Dianne said he was told that his sight was "excellent".

10.07 pm   Went to the uni today to meet the two professors I know in economics and finance with Jack and Dianne. Jack is ready to go back to uni (hallelujah!) and he was on point and on song. Did not miss a beat. Knew exactly what he wanted, and he lead the conversation. In a nutshell Mardi and Sree said they will do whatever it takes to get him back and help with any issue – door is always open. Lovely people. We have all had an extra bounce in our step since.

Aiming to get him back in Semester 2, July this year.

WhatsApp POST

7 April   But I have a request. Could someone find out for me the laws regarding driving a car with a "malignant" brain tumour? Jack has just left his neurosurgeon who said he cannot ever drive again while he has a malignant brain tumour. His oncologist has a different view. Jack pretty upset so looking for any comprehensive advice … Maybe it is State-based? However, Jack was undergoing testing at the behest of his oncologist (eyes and neurology to review sequence of seizures). Not sure if it is universal, State-based and if so, is there discretion (such as a recommendation from his clinicians?)?

We (Jack, Dianne and I) met with his oncologists today (which now includes John as well as Rosie) and it was suggested to reintroduce temozolomide, combined with lomustine as more effective against paediatric GBM.

Observation after this and collated over several weeks (in my notes): Again, reasonably well tolerated by Jack in first two weeks, but more tired, and needs sleeps in daytime. Appetite reduced, but no nausea.

WhatsApp POST   7.14 pm

Jack starts his next dose of chemo tonight. I hate these nights. Anyway, just ordered pizza so he has something to look forward to.

He slept well after his new 'cocktail' chemo dose. Took a sleeping pill just in case and slept peacefully through the night. Just had breakfast and now joking with Hugh. Whew.

Incidentally the State Attorney General just diagnosed with "aggressive, malignant brain tumours" (several in fact) and I suspect glioblastoma. She had been told that she has a very short time left. 43.   10.50 am

Maybe I'm just tuned into brain cancer now, but the beast seems to be on the rise. Is Jack on new chemo regime?   11.01 am

Yes and no. Temozolomide is what he was originally on and lomustine is what he has been on since January. Because the theory is that he has paediatric GBM there is evidence that combining them can be more effective. 1+1=3 theory. We will know in the next 4-6 weeks. Paediatric GBM tumours do not respond well to temozolomide alone. And the fact it did not respond leads to the theory that he has a paediatric tumour, which usually does not respond to standard (temozolomide) treatment.

9 April Orthoptist/Ophthalmology check-up. Showed improved fields, but in bottom right quadrant a "small dead zone" remained. Ophthalmologist happy with health of his eyes and advised Jack's vision is on right path to consider return to driving after another review in July.

Access to ABT414 granted on compassionate grounds. Advised that it can be administered with the current lomustine/temozolomide cocktail but have agreed to monitor success (or otherwise) of current cocktail alone and not add ABT414 (or even replace current cocktail) unless there are obvious signs that current chemo is not working.

14 April Just had a good chat to Jack. First two days of chemo were a bit of a struggle. Day 3 was OK and the final two days a walk in the park. He finished Tuesday and is in good spirits. Laughing, talking about a string of social and political issues which he identifies with. Dianne and I are very liberally minded and have brought the boys up with open

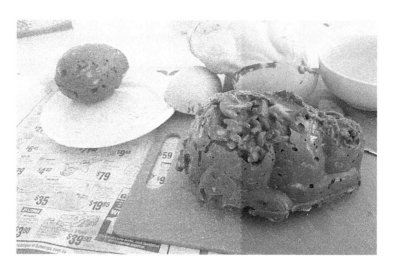

Jack's homemade Easter egg!

minds and encouraged them to embrace humanity with all its preferences, whether they be religious, sexual or gender based. Treat everyone equally. Jack has always been the most vocal and opinionated in expressing his (similar) views. He is also young and like most young people he rages against institutional and generational bias.

He is not having much dinner so as he can hit his Easter egg hard tonight.

When he is like this it is almost like nothing has happened. And we can pretend that this is the way it will be forever. So, a lousy Christmas but Easter is shaping up well.

WhatsApp POST

Jack has been offered access to ABT414 on "compassionate grounds". He has strong receptor characteristics of EGF in his tumour as identified by our good Sydney professors. Thus, he is a natural candidate. This is our plan C alongside Garvan.

Lining up the ducks. I had a terrible argument with him tonight which showed me how much of the old Jack has returned. It was ugly, but we kissed and made up.

Ironically, we would have clashed regardless of his illness as I was the provocateur and sometimes, in all relationships, partners clash as was the case this night. Dianne irritated me while we were playing a game and I walked away and said I didn't want to play anymore. Jack, typically (always taking his mother's side regardless of the circumstances), verbally tore into me. I got angry and defended myself and told him sometimes people have arguments but, in most cases, it is none of your business and this "is between Mum and I, not you, so butt out!".

It took several days of tension and Dianne acting as the peacemaker to finally get Jack and I in the same room to discuss. The chemistry between two people is complex as are the interactions and I did my best to explain why I lost my cool and abruptly left the game. But I also opened up a little too much and Matthew, who was listening to the discourse between Jack, Dianne and myself, got upset, as he probably hadn't heard me speak so openly about Dianne. Anyway, after I had exhausted the subject and again accused Jack of preferring his Mum over me, he looked at me, smiled and then gave me a big hug.

WhatsApp POST

30 April   Yes. The best I have seen him although a little wary about saying that given the same comments I made just prior to Christmas.

He was out with friends last night and did not get home till just after 1.

Seeing Garvan in Sydney on 12 May. He is hoping to also be allowed to drive again but needs to be cleared by a neurologist. That appointment is in June.

But laughing, joking and arguing and sometimes his old prickly self.

MAY
2 May   **email MICHAEL BUCKLAND ▸ KF**

Hi Ken

The assay did identify some potential new pathways for treatment via current clinical trials. They are all theoretical options rather than proven treatments, and they may end up being prohibitively expensive or unsuitable for Jack.

The appropriateness of any given clinical trial is something
I can't comment on with any expertise. That is why you will
need to liaise with oncologists that are knowledgeable in these
areas. There will be no 'right' answer in any of this – it will be a
choice for you and Jack working with the oncologists, and your
eventual conclusion may be that the best option is to do nothing
else for now. I would suggest sending the report around to a
few oncologists including David Thomas, Mustafa Khasraw and
David Ziegler and get their opinions on the best way forward.
I am working to get the patient identifiers on the report –
ironically it seems just as hard as doing the assay. As soon as I
have this I will send it through to your nominated oncologists

It has been a good experience for us to try out this new assay,
and I am learning a lot not only about the technical aspects
but also the practical issues of delineating management
pathways with oncologists. So you certainly don't owe us
anything at all. I will be in touch again shortly.

All the best

Michael

MICHAEL BUCKLAND

Royal Prince Alfred Hospital

Met with Dr Subo at Garvan Institute in Sydney Dr Subo said **12 May**
that Jack was eligible for the MoST Programme although final
eligibility will depend on key markers found in his tumour. If these
were not present – that is markers that can be targets for specific
treatments/drugs – then Garvan could not assist Jack. We were told
that testing for these markers could take up to "8 weeks".

WhatsApp POSTS

9.48 pm   *Fantastic news. I was sweating on hearing.*

9.51 pm   Slept on the plane. He was completely out of it. Not used to getting up at 4.30. But when he woke up started playing chess on his phone. Wow I thought. Where have you been hiding!!

9.54 pm   Checking dates: he is 12 months on 8 July. He is 14 months on 8 September. Pass those two dates and alive he is Mr 5% and we are in uncharted territory.

9.55 pm   *On good track. Well done.*

10.05 pm   So I wonder, with three deaths that I am aware of recently (23 year old woman dead 10 months after diagnosis; 12 year old girl dead after 10 months; 26 year old man dead after 16 months) how much time do we have really? I am kidding myself if I say forever. It is a platitude. So, no nice words please. He won't make it. How much time do we have? How much. No need to answer because I know you don't know but nothing I know can stop this ultimate death sentence. I am not good with 5% and that is where he will sit at 16 months. But can he REALLY get to 16 months? 5% make it that far. 5%. 5%. 5%.

10.18 pm   OK. But no God, because as an atheist (as is Jack) prayers and praying are not doing it. Medical science and probability we can back. Divine intervention won't work as there is no Santa Claus and the Easter Bunny is a nice kiddies story.

10.18 pm   *Didn't mention faith.*

10.21 pm   I know sorry, but I have so many friends praying so was making a BIG statement as feeling low, low low at the moment. Wasn't to you. Just talking so sorry, wasn't meant to be personal.

10.23 pm   *No. Didn't take it personally. But sticking with the information at hand. Let your friends pray. Hedge your bets!*

But Jack said to Dianne the other day he actually is thinking   10.25 pm
now he will survive. First time as he was accepting prior to
that his early death. Yes, day by day. Day by fucking day.

It is as if a little afraid to dare think of a positive   10.30 pm
outcome. Keeping yourself from hoping

Now into the sake. Hope Japanese rice wine will change my   10.34 pm
demeanour as not healthy at the moment.

But didn't you hear today some hope?   10.35 pm

We have hope in the plan we have re treatments. Today is   10.41 pm
about more treatments. My back up plan. And that is what I am
good at – finding solutions. And this is another possible option.
But this disease takes no prisoners and there is no magic
bullet. The statistics are against Jack and 95% of GBM patients
are dead at 16 months. So, news today is that we may be able
to help but there is no cure and it may just buy him time.

Not 100%??   10.42 pm

No. But given the shit we have gone through why would Jack   10.48 pm
be a survivor and amongst the 5%?? Sorry sake kicking in and
feeling cynical and lost. Just shit scared and not sure how to
deal with this reality.

No, on second thought, I can work with 5%. He has been a lot   **13 May**
of fun today so if 5% is all I got then we will roll the dice Choo
Choo and keep playing.

Forgot to add that I also asked Dr Subo (Garvan) whether
there were many patients of Jack's age that she was seeing.
Her response was sobering as she said, "Yes, quite a lot. Too
many actually …" There were at least five cases she knew
of that were ahead of Jack by only a couple of weeks and

16 May   all around his age. She also said, "seeing a lot of sarcomas amongst young people and many of which are untreatable" and thus almost always fatal.

They also asked if Dianne and I would agree to "gene testing" (mapping our whole genome). I said yes in the name of science but also answered "no" for the question that asked if I wanted to be told if they found some gene defect that could cause cancer etc., etc. in future years. Dianne in agreement. We have enough to worry about as it is and don't have time to worry about our own mortality. Stefan was bad enough with his motor bike (I used to ring every time there was a fatality near him which he always thought was amusing); Adrian in the jungles of Peru (or other parts of South America where civil rights are alien – I made sure he got the top travel insurance which covered kidnapping [one of my great fears]) and now Jack. Parenting sucks. Hugh had a headache the other day and some loss of vision yesterday. And you can't half guess what Dianne and I were thinking last night … Whisky tonight!!!

19 May   On 19 May met with Jack's oncologist. Meeting was brief, as Jack had no issues to discuss. Started his five-day cycle that night (two nights with lomustine and temozolomide) and three more nights on temozolomide, finishing on 23 May. No ill effects.

WhatsApp POSTS

21 May   Day 2 done. Slept well, no side effects. One of the professors at the Uni inquired about Jack on Friday and said they will send him his course outline for semester 2 soon. He is looking forward to going back. Starts in July. On 8 July he is one-year post diagnosis and beyond that in the 10% still alive post diagnosis.

23 May

This is Day 5 and then end of the cycle. 5 days, not 6. 5.58 am

Current cycle that is. Start again in 6 weeks 5.59 am

Jack had another good night. Finishes tonight. Dianne cooking 10.55 am
bacon and eggs for a hungry boy as I write this. Such a relief.
After surgery and the dexamethasone really stuffed him up.
This is a walk in the park by comparison. No dex, just hard
drugs. Takes me back to the '60s …

31 May

95% dead at 16 months. 90% after 12-14 months. He was told 5.32 pm
on 8 July last year he had 12 months. Must beat that curse.
16 months I have 4 months more than I thought I had.
4 months is better than nothing. Forever is better than
anything but unless you believe in fairies, God and Santa
Clause he won't make it. If I get him to his 21st on
25 November, then Dianne and I will be the happiest couple in
history. We have hopes but we are also realistic.

OK 25 Nov is a nice date to aim for … or beyond XX 5.34 pm

Yes, 12-year-old's family completely devastated. At 5.48 pm
least we got another 8 years with Jack. I have told him
that story and he has told me others of similar young
tragedies. He reads this stuff all the time and knows his
time is limited.

When we were coming home from Sydney after Garvan there
was a boy (reckon 8?) who was bald, sallow face, dark eyes. I

thought leukemia but didn't say anything to Jack. Jack pulled me aside as we were going through security and said did you see that boy? I said yes and he smiled and said, "It could be worse Dad".

JUNE

6 June WhatsApp POST

Just a quick update. Jack good and no adverse changes since last post. Next MRI is on 19 June and we will know where we sit then and decide on more of the same or change course. However, the situation is having a marked and adverse impact on Hugh who spent most of Sunday in tears, not eating and not coming out of his room. He has been (seemingly) pretty resilient up until now with Chris being the one to feel the emotional burden but it caught up with Hugh on Sunday. He woke up and started thinking about Jack and then went down a rabbit hole and not resurfaced. That "depression" (and that is what it is according to his Dr) then morphed into a dark journey across all the (his view) fragile aspects of his life, like failing in his studies, not getting sufficient ATAR points to get into medicine and breaking up with his girlfriend. All of which are unfounded but in his fragile state he is inconsolable.

Dianne and I spoke to Jack and he spent some time with Hugh last night talking one-on-one. We saw this fragile emotional state once before after he watched a movie, which unhinged him for about two weeks. He was so upset it scared us big time. We hope between Chris (who is paying extra attention to him), Jack, Dianne and I we can see that cheeky little boy back in our lives soon. Have kept Matthew out of it for the moment as he has exams to focus on.

As I review this observation now (15 months on) and discussions I had with my family regarding all that we were experiencing as a family, there was a lot of hidden pain the boys were feeling which every so often would emerge and then quickly disappear. But I think the overriding strength that the family drew on was my ongoing monologue regarding new research and/or people I had spoken to that gave us hope. I was always talking about something that I had discovered; some new information I had uncovered; a new clinical trial; or feedback from clinicians. My patter was upbeat publicly but privately I had monumental doubts and many times when alone I would crumple and that feeling of despair would be all-consuming.

And I think my role was more pivotal than Dianne's in this vein as she was doing all the heavy lifting while encouraging me to continue pursuing, researching and talking to anyone that might offer us more time. It was a practical division of labour as we had three younger boys (all three in high school) and Jack needed constant care and all of that was a full-time job, which Dianne embraced. She said to me, "You are good at this, so just keep doing it". I remember being quite chuffed but on refection now, if I was so good at it, how come Jack died?

WhatsApp POSTS

Jack MRI tomorrow at 8 45. He is nervous. Big test this one.　　**18 June**
Get results at end of week when we meet oncologist.

Andrew Hunn rang:

"Continued shrinkage/contraction of previously identified 'tumour'　　**20 June**
area". That is clearly positive. However, have identified new area of
enhancement in the splenium. Don't know what this is and could
be a new area of tumour or equally possible impact of radiation.
Overall, he said "it appears the current treatment is working."

115

Good result considering. Not perfect but could be worse. Jack has no excuse not to enrol for second semester now. None, zip, zero.

Di read a bit about the splenium and it is common for lesions in this area after radiation therapy.

I know we are spinning this but what if it is exactly that and not more tumour growth? And the neurosurgeon who is usually pretty blunt and sees tumours everywhere, was giving the radiation theory a lot of credibility. Maybe, just maybe, we won this round with a clear knockout …?

Jack smiling. "Told you so." Bastard.

2:55 pm   *Love that kid X*

23 June   In 2016, I joined an online GBM support group. During that time, I posted a narrative on Jack. I got many responses. This is just one:

ONLINE GBM SUPPORT GROUP

Thank you Ken for sharing Jack's story. It is so inspiring that Jack did not give up and he is doing well!

We have a 21-year-old son fighting GBM too. He was diagnosed 15 months ago when he was still 19. It started with a grand mal seizure, and all the up and down similar to yours. He did the radiation, 6 months TMZ, and then we put him on a bunch of re-purposed medication and supplements and CBD+THC. His MRI is clear so far. He just graduated from college a couple weeks ago.

There is a book called "Anticancer, A New Way of Life" by Dave Servan-Schreiber. You must read it. There is also this documentary: https://www.survivingterminalcancer.com/

Not many parents have to endure what we have gone through. Please keep us posted on how Jack is doing. Our best wishes to Jack and your family!

Holly

ARSENAL   29 June

As I have noted earlier, we were a fanatical English Football League (EPL) family and Jack, Chris and Adrian were Arsenal tragics. With the prognosis for Jack being dour we all thought Jack would never see his team play live as it was one of his lifetime passions to see an actual game in Europe. But before Jack was diagnosed, Arsenal announced that it would be playing some friendly matches in Sydney in July 2017 and the boys had previously arranged to buy tickets when they came on sale. And they came on sale while Jack was recovering at Calvary Hospital from his first major brain surgery. At that time, I wrote to Arsenal explaining Jack's diagnosis and asked if Jack could meet the team when visiting Australia.

WhatsApp POST

Adrian, Jack, Chris and Hugh have been invited to the team party and training session. See below. Jack will be thrilled. Waiting for him to wake up.

email ANDREW PIGOTT, Arsenal FC ▶ KF

Good afternoon,

I hope this email finds you well.

You contacted the Arsenal club some time ago and my colleague Mark has possibly been in touch with you since.

We are very excited about our visit to Australia this summer and would like to invite you to the official tour fan party event we have organised on Friday 14th July. This will be located at the ANZ Stadium with doors opening at 2 pm.

I have organised x4 Golden Circle tickets for you at the event. Your wristbands can be collected from myself on the day from Box Office J/K between 1.30 pm-2 pm. There will be no collections available after this time for the golden circle.

You can then access the event via Gate K or Gate M from 2 pm. The fan event will start at 2:30 pm with appearances from members of the 1st team, Club legend, Gunnersaurus. Following the fan party there will be an open training session that the full 1st team will participate in. The event should finish by 6:30 pm.

In the meantime, please can you confirm you are able to attend the event and provide me with the best contact number for yourself should I need to reach you on the day?

Kind regards

Andrew Pigott

Travel, Events and Supporter Liaison

Arsenal Football Club

Highbury House I 75 Drayton Park I London I N5 1BU

Jack was pleased (and that is the best word I can use to explain his reaction as he was never one to show too much emotion). In hindsight though I think he got the biggest buzz from the reaction of his brothers and friends as they were clearly very impressed and I suspect he got a lot of traffic on his Facebook account.

JUNE NOTES

These Notes, like most of the other Notes I have included in this book were records in part maintained by Dianne. She kept a diary of his appointments, treatments, prescriptions and medications as well as any medical issues and I kept a log on his wellbeing (making my own observations daily). I would merge Dianne's Notes with my own (filtering out any duplication) so that we had a running collective on all things Jack. We did this for several reasons but I also thought if by some bizarre miracle, Jack survived, these Notes could provide some insight that may help others. I was always a dreamer.

Neuropsychologist follow up on 22 June, provided Jack with some interesting findings re progress of brain function. The report suggested Jack had made only minor improvements in some key areas, however Jack disputes this and considers he has improved greatly. Not sure if he will bother with another follow-up, none scheduled. But all three of us – Jack, Dianne and myself – knew Jack was not the same and I feared (but never voiced although Dianne was less in denial than I was) some of the damage to his brain was irreversible. I told Jack many times, let me fix the cancer and I will fix everything else.

His visit with Dr Lucie Aldous, neurologist on 27 June, was very positive. She went through his history and recommended continuation of current meds for at least another three months. At which time she thought he would be OK to start driving again, as long as no seizures occur.

Orthoptist/Ophthalmology was postponed till 14 September to coincide with next Neurology appointment regarding his application to get driver's licence back.

JULY

5 July   **WhatsApp POST**

5:10 pm   Jack's platelets are very low and have been falling. Having a platelet transfusion tomorrow.

5:20 pm   *Nothing more than side effects chemo?*

5:21 pm   Suspect so. Not sure.

12 July   Jack wanted a tattoo but because he was on chemo he couldn't have one. Thus, I bought some temporary tattoos with the date 8 July 2017 which represented one year after his diagnosis. However, Jack wanted the date of his diagnosis – 8 July 2016. I stuffed up but he forgave me.

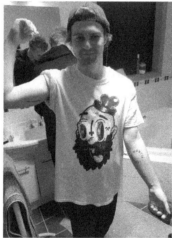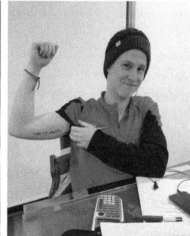

Jack, left, and Chris

14 July   Jack went to see Arsenal in Sydney with Adrian, Chris and Hugh. The passes that Arsenal afforded allowed both Chris and Jack in to meet the players. This was very special as very few of these passes were handed out.

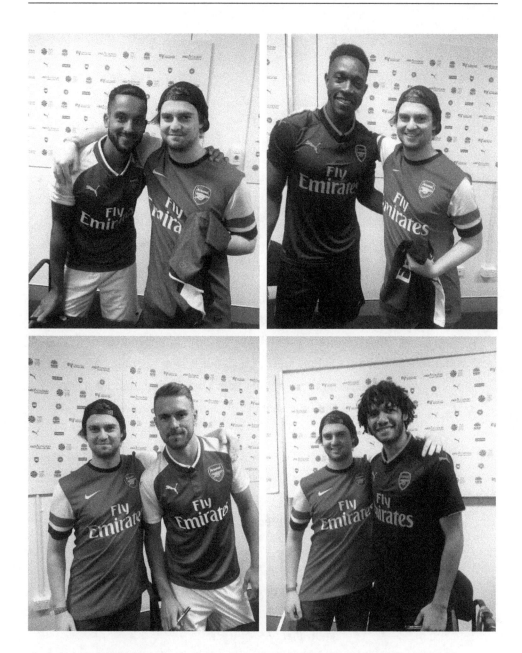

Jack with Arsenal players. clockwise from top left, Theo Walcott, Danny Welbeck, Mohammed Elneny and Aaron Ramsey

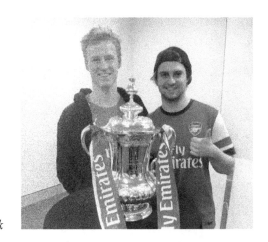

Chris and Jack

Some correspondence between Jack and I last night (below). It followed a good chat about life and living. He knows his chances are small and said, "Dad I know all the statistics and they are not good and know I may not have long". He said he did not hold out much hope, but it won't get him down and he is prepared to accept his fate. I dwelled on that for a couple of minutes and then shot off my email. His response is as below.

16 July
9.39 pm

K I got you in to meet the Arsenal team; I got you a slot at Garvan; I got your result in Investment Analysis changed from an F to a HD; and I got the university doing backflips in the Economics department to have you back and make sure you do well so why can't I lick this disease? Why?

> **J** *Haha you're killing it!!*
> *Thanks for everything you do for me dad, I love you, as always. No matter the circumstances I want you to know that I AM HAPPY.*
> *Not many people can have what I have and be happy with their life as I am.*

With Jack it was always hard to read his emotions as he showed very little and just got on with life. This demeanour continued after he was diagnosed so I had no reason to suspect that he wasn't happy with his life. I just don't know what he was thinking other than he thought I would somehow find a way out of this maze – as did everyone – as I was always discovering new people and research and I would discuss every positive bit of information with him and anyone else who would listen. I maintained this spirited monologue and even words and phrases I would take out of context and add my own (positive) interpretation. I wasn't deliberately trying to be misleading but I could find a silver lining in anything I read or any conversation I had because I had to; because if I didn't I would go mad. Curl up in a foetal position and die. I think Dianne was sometimes sceptical and she was sometimes less hopeful than I was and then again there were times when we thought we had a shot.

WhatsApp POSTS

Jack's platelets have dipped a little but only modestly, although his white blood cell count is low. On Friday it will be 8 weeks since last chemo session (cycle is every 6 weeks). Oncologist said not to start now and meeting on Friday. I spoke to Garvan and was told another 2-3 weeks at least to complete testing. Thereafter his results are put to a panel of specialists and a tailored solution to treat his tumour recommended. It is also possible that he may not be eligible for treatment at Garvan but think that is unlikely. Thus, between a rock and hard place. Don't want to lose recent momentum and waiting that long could be problematic. He has another blood test tomorrow and that may give us a lead – blood count good so start lomustine/temozolomide course or consider waiting on other option/s. The only other

19 July
1.37 pm

option we have here is Hobart is ABT414 (http://www.cancernetwork.com/sno-2016/abt-414-shows-promise-against-egfr-amplified-gbm). Jack has high level of EGFR expression in his tumour (as discovered by the two Sydney professors).

Jack very well at the moment so in a good place but that can change quickly. Currently talking to Hugh who is pretty messed up over his relationship with his girlfriend, plus Jack. Today we had a breakthrough and finally he gave us some answers: he wants to break up but doesn't know how to tell her given the almost inseparable relationship they have had over the last 12 months. It is guilt and that has led to depression. He was in a very bad way this morning but finally, finally (!) we have an answer!!

Parenting sucks. I am going to come back as an alcoholic eunuch!

22 July OK update. Jack the best he has ever been. Touch wood. Said in the meeting with the oncologist yesterday that he approached returning to Uni with some trepidation but said he found he was "300% better" than he thought was possible. No headaches and no problems reading. Plus remembering everything. His white blood cell count is low (but not a concern) and his platelets are improving but not sufficiently high enough for his next dose of chemo, so we are in a holding pattern. We discussed ABT414 but again he needs his platelets closer to 100+ (at the moment they have reading of 69). As previously noted, Garvan is several weeks away and I gave his oncologist an update. If his blood count improves, probably have another (less potent) dose of temozolomide/ lomustine.

11.34 pm Listening to Jack, Hugh and Chris argue (nicely) over football. Almost normal.

Nice. 11.35 pm

Watching Arsenal vs Chelsea live. Di there too stirring the pot. 11.36 pm
I can almost dream that this is the way it should be.

It is the way it is 11.36 pm

Jack narky and so provocative. So so Jack. 11.37 pm

Sitting here with Jack helping him with his economics **25 July**
homework. He is so back!!! I almost think I have woken from a
bad dream.

JULY NOTES

Jack was due to start his next round of lomustine/temozolomide for six weeks on 30 June, but his platelets were too low and subsequent weekly blood tests showed they continued to fall (to "17").

He had a platelet transfusion on 7 July and the levels remained elevated, allowing him to travel to Sydney for Arsenal matches (13-16 July). In his meeting with his oncologists on 21 July it was not recommended that he start his new course of lomustine/temozolomide until his platelets were at (or above) "100". We also discussed Garvan (see next point) and ABT414 but it was recommended that he not consider ABT414 until his platelets were closer to (or above) 100. Next blood test scheduled for 25 July.

"Emily" rang from Garvan on Monday, 17 July to say that it would be at least another three weeks before the testing of Jack's tumour would be completed. At that time the results would be put in front of a group of specialists who will then recommend a "tailored" solution for Jack.

AUGUST

7 August

11:17 am

UPDATE: Jack's blood count was back to normal last week so started his final chemo dose on Friday. Final in the sense that lomustine has serious long-term effects (such as permanent platelet count loss) so usually patients have four doses (maximum). This is Jack's fourth. Again, no side effects other than extreme tiredness.

Next stage will be (and following his next MRI for later this month) ABT414, Garvan or do nothing if the MRI result is clear. He is also back at Uni and studying 8-10 hours a day and 7 days a week. This is the way he always was and the only difference this time is that his brain function is compromised and comprehension and short-term memory are challenged. He had an online quiz the other night in financial mathematics and I sat with him. The first question I disagreed with his answer and two more questions he struggled with basic comprehension. And I do mean basic. The rest he whizzed through and didn't need my counsel. His score was 9/10 and when he went back to Q1 he realised the mistake he had made which was all good. However, in relation to the other two questions he had a mental blank. The next day Dianne said he got very upset as he was starting to realise he is not the same anymore and he will never get a job. A rare moment of emotion for Jack.

Fast forward to last night. Same deal. I sat with my calculator and spreadsheets and did all the questions and then Jack would check with me to see if we agreed. In all but one we disagreed. He then explained to me my error. He was right. This time he got 100% and it was ALL his own work. The relief on his face was palpable. Baby steps.

Should say that in all but one we agreed. I had a lesson in humility but well deserved!

He is, no matter what we say or do still a high achiever. This is the way he has always been: 8-10 hours a day and 7 days a week. And there is nothing we can say or do that can change that.

10 August

Jack is dropping Macro. Had the test today and needs twice as long as normal students (which the Uni usually caters for) but he wasn't given any extra time or assistance. He has trouble reading and comprehension/processing is slow, and he was completely lost today. Too stressed out and the fact that he has is back at Uni is a miracle in itself but there is a danger in over doing it.

Di reckons Jack was worried, but I didn't see it. Then again, she is with him all day. He has not had any symptoms that would concern me – like severe headaches. He gets slight headaches but that has always been the case and that cycle hasn't changed. Also, he is now spending a lot of time reading since returning to Uni and his eyes and general eyesight are not good and he gets tired easily, which would explain the headaches.

18 August

Re-reading this note again it is representative of many conversations that I had with Dianne – she would always call it the way she saw it and I typically would be in denial. With Dianne the glass was always half empty but with me at this time, it was half full. She was the more pragmatic one and made her own honest (and sometimes brutally honest) observations and I would ignore it if it didn't fit my thematic. It was never a cause for an argument but a discussion. Dianne and I are naturally combative people so we had a lot of reasons to engage in an argument but never about Jack during this time.

22 August   MRI showed no sign of growth in area identified in January (good thing) and a very small increase in new area identified in last MRI. Hard to know what it all means as Jack delayed his last chemo session due to low blood count and recent chemo is still working its way through his system. Meeting oncologist on Friday. Rang Garvan yesterday and left a VM but not heard back. Jack worried but I think that is misplaced. All in all, I would say a positive result.

25 August   Just left Oncology. The news is bad. The new site (which is now confirmed as tumour) is growing quickly and it is inoperable. On the plus he has been accepted into the MoST programme and there are a number of experimental (although immunotherapy based) treatments that he is eligible for. Secondly, we have been asked to consider more (but highly specialised) radiation treatment (in Melbourne). This is an interim measure and may give us more time. Third there is ABT414 (immunotherapy as well) available here in Hobart. Finally, there is the do nothing and die gracefully.

Dianne and I are looking at everything and Jack just wants some advice.

28 August   I keep notes on Jack so that I have a running history:

On Monday 28 August, I got a call from Dr Subo Thavaneswaran (Garvan Institute) and she answered all my outstanding questions:

If Jack accepted treatment at the Garvan, each cycle would take 5-6 hours at a time and be repeated once a month. Side effects are minimal but could include skin rash, fatigue and diarrhoea. Possible more serious side effects include irritation of the lining of the lungs and/or colitis. Side effects, MRI and blood tests could be coordinated through Hobart Royal. MRI's would be scheduled for every 8 weeks after every second cycle;

On the ABT414 vs the cocktail of immunotherapy drugs (combination of Durvalumab + Tremelimumab) recommended for Jack, she said (think I have this correct?):

- Jack did not have an IDH mutation (that is his GBM was primary and did not develop from a lower grade tumour), thus Durvalumab + Tremelimumab may not be as effective as a targeted drug, like ABT414;

- She confirmed that Garvan had identified the high level of EGFR expression in Jack's tumour (originally discovered by Sydney University) and felt that the targeted approach would be preferable (that is ABT414 in favour of immunotherapy) as the Garvan cocktail was not targeted and its effectiveness against primary GBM is unproven;

- ABT414 has some proven success against GBM;

- In discussions with other clinicians, it was broadly agreed that ABT414 would be recommended over Durvalumab + Tremelimumab (that is "targeted" preferred to "non-targeted");

- Jack would still be eligible to access the treatment offered by Garvan in the event that ABT414 was not effective in his treatment. However, she did remark that Garvan had just "64 spots available" for treatment using Durvalumab + Tremelimumab, although had requested additional access to the drugs. Nonetheless, Jack would still be accepted.

I spoke to Victoria and told her what Subo had told me and that we would go with ABT414 here in Hobart, although I was anxious to understand what Dr Michael Dally has advised in regard to possible radiation treatment in Melbourne for Jack. The advice from Michael was that where the tumour was located, the risks of harm to Jack (particularly on his right side) outweighed any possible benefit he might receive from the treatment.

Victoria confirmed that the ABT414 will be available for Jack next Monday, 4 September.

Jack's oncologist rang at 4 pm today; agreed with everything that Subo had stated re ABT414:

1. ABT414 has been ordered and hopefully it will be ready to be administered on Monday 4 September. Any slippage will mean an appointment for Jack later in the week. We will be notified of time later this week;

2. The drug works very quickly – within "hours" – attaching itself to the EGFR cells and then "uncoupling and delivering its bomb";

3. He needs to take eye drops two days before the treatment and 5 days after. The drops have been ordered and we should expect a call from the pharmacist any day now;

4. He will need to put aside 3-4 hours on Monday with one of his parents there to have a meeting to discuss side effects;

5. The lomustine is no longer having an impact as his blood counts are back to normal;

6. Can get access to some immunotherapy drugs also such as pembrolizumab (provided by Keytruda). Access to tremelimumab is problematic in Australia (at the moment).

AUGUST NOTES

Jack's bloods finally recovered to normal on 2 August and commenced a reduced lomustine dose of 80mg but same dose 140mg temozolomide. No adverse side effects so far (8 August), except tiredness, mild nausea. Reduced appetite, but still eating healthy meals, though reduced in size.

Blood test week ending Friday 18 August showed good results.

MRI on 18 August.

Meeting with John and Rosie on 25 August was confronting. The new area earlier identified had grown quickly since the last MRI but was inoperable. It was recommended that we consider a review of Jack's tumour by Dr Michael Dally, Radiation Oncologist at Epworth (not Peter Mac). Reason being that the tumour is growing in a sensitive (and inoperable) part of his brain and this may need to be addressed quickly before it causes some "severe neurological problems" and in advance of any further treatment. The term used was (we recall?) "stereotactic radiosurgery" (or something like that).

I responded to Garvan ("Emily") on 29 August, advising that we would not be accepting its offer to treat Jack at this stage as we will be opting for ABT414 in Hobart, following Subo's advice. However, confirmed that we may need to revisit this offer in the event that the ABT414 is not helpful.

Jack's annual Audiologist appointment on 28 August, showed no change to his hearing.

SEPTEMBER

2 September   Also, been in touch with a couple of Jack's mates and they are looking after him. He is going out again tonight. Hoping for Tuesday access to ABT414 and he starts the eye drops tomorrow. I am very hopeful, as this drug has delivered some incredible results on a few GBM sufferers although it doesn't work for everyone.

4 September   There has been some delay in getting the ABT414 drug to Hobart but unavoidable. However, he is already getting some symptoms of pressure from the tumour and we need to hit it now and hit it hard. Nothing we can do though but just watch him every minute. No one is currently on it in Hobart so Jack is very special, but delays can be fatal.

Yes, but a lot counting on the efficacy of the ABT414. Could be a magic bullet and then again, not. He also dropped his last subject at Uni today. This is too much for him at the moment and I need him de-stressed. It was an easy decision for him.

8 September   14 months today. ABT414 at 2 pm at the Royal today.

12 September   Have locked in Jack Greene (bar in Salamanca) for Jack's 21st on 25 November.

Also had some correspondence with Olivia Newton-John Cancer Research Institute yesterday regarding clinical work being undertaken there in relation to brain cancer. Was informed that the therapy Jack is using now, ABT414, is "it" (current state of play and the one that is showing the most promise). There is a clinical trial starting later this year (which is interesting as we are [unusually] already in the queue and have launched!), but good feedback.

	17 September
And radiotherapy?	12:08 am

No too dangerous. The radiologist said he can have a shot, but good chance Jack would be a vegetable. Doors closing — 12:11 am

But others opening — 12.12 am

Time is against us though. If this thing continues to grow we are only left with experimental drugs as surgery and radiology ruled out — 12.14 am

OK … right at this moment he sounds to be doing OK — 12.25 am

Better day today. May have dodged a bullet — 7.00 pm

Di just left oncologist and called. Jack getting his second dose of ABT414 now. News is (surprisingly) all good. All of Jack's symptoms – near seizure like moments, headaches and worsening eyesight are all related to the drug and very doubtful any of the adverse signs are tumour related. Oncologist said that as the drugs kills the cancer cells it upsets the brain balance resulting in swelling etc. and that is what is expected of the ABT414 so she is quite happy with how Jack has responded. Platelets are a little low and liver result less than perfect but nothing to be concerned about. Next MRI will be in about 6 weeks. — **22 September**

How is Jack feeling himself? Is he having the odd drink? — 1.12 pm
I am overdue to send something silly x

Funny you ask. About 8 o'clock last night Matt came up and asked if he could have a whisky and I said yes. Five minutes later Jack came out of his room and asked the same question and I — 1.19 pm said YES! YES! YES!!! He has had fantastic sleeps the last two nights but the loss of (and blurred) vision he finds very frustrating. That said, sometimes it comes back, and it is perfect.

1.31 pm   Kate thanks, but there is nothing I can think of other than a bottle of whisky for Jack, with the note "To drink on your 21st or when you are cancer free, whatever comes first!". I am also wary about lauding these moments as we may have won one battle (and that is not absolutely for certain, only one opinion) but we are a long way from winning the war. If this though gives him six months before we need to think about our next steps, we are six months into the path of a range of other treatments that are currently being developed, such as related to the malaria and polio vaccines.

1.33 pm   I don't now look at keeping him alive indefinitely but in six-month increments as it allows me time to work on (and execute) my next play.

25 September

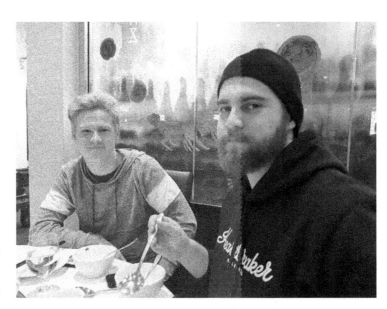

Chris and Jack back at Me Wah, again

SEPTEMBER NOTES

Jack had his first infusion of ABT414 on the afternoon of 8 September. There were no adverse side effects. Prior to that – on Wednesday 6 September – he started the eye drops to avoid any "eye" problems that have been identified in earlier patients taking ABT414.

On or about 12 September he noted that his peripheral vision on his right side was very poor. On 14 September, Jack had his scheduled Ophthalmology RHH appointment. Fields on right side had significantly deteriorated and obviously driving is not permitted. More importantly, his eyes had no effects from ABT414 – nerves etc. Look great. To be reviewed again in three months.

On Friday – one week later – 15 September Dianne rang me and said Jack was not good. He has an increasing incidence of headaches and felt borderline seizure "auras". The next day, Saturday, he was worse. Panadol has been the medication of choice although Jack says he does not believe that it makes any difference. He eventually took 4mg of dexamethasone (which he hates as it effects his bowels and sleep patterns) and later that afternoon one Endone tablet. Early evening, he said the Endone did not have any effect and his headache was worsening ("4 out of 10"). We thought it was possible that we may have to get Jack to hospital to access morphine if the headache pain increased. Later that night he came up from his room and said that he was a lot better. The pain had eased substantially and he felt fine. I fell asleep on the couch and was woken by Jack at 4.30 am. He had a smile on his face and said he felt fine but couldn't sleep.

On Sunday he was a lot better – didn't take any dexamethasone and didn't need any Endone.

On Monday 18 September, Jack played futsal with his friends in a Monday night competition. He had poor vision and claimed that he couldn't see but he did bloody well and a lot of the old skills were apparent. However, he exhausted quickly as unfit and the compartment syndrome problems in his calves re-emerged. He played 15-20 minutes though and this old man was impressed.

On 22 September, Jack had his second dose of ABT414. At the meeting his oncologist remarked that all his symptoms were classic ABT414 and didn't think they were cancer related.

He played futsal again on Monday 25 September and again despite his calve pain and unfitness, did bloody well again.

Last week (and particularly Saturday and Sunday 30 September/1 October) Jack experienced a range of symptoms – severe tiredness, poor vision, sore eyes and sensitivity to light. Also, not sleeping well. Again, all classic symptoms of ABT414 (http://www.cancerresearchuk.org/about-cancer/find-a-clinical-trial/a-trial-of-abt-414-for-glioblastoma-that-has-come-back-intellance-2#undefined).

OCTOBER

1 October   Jack not bad considering, although suffering a range of standard side effects of the treatment. I sent him the list below and he smiled and said, "yep I got every one of them". It is his blurred vision which is the most debilitating and he looks like he is going to sleep sometimes when he is sitting at the table as he just shuts his eyes and doesn't move.

http://www.cancerresearchuk.org/about-cancer/find-a-clinical-trial/a-trial-of-abt-414-for-glioblastoma-that-has-come-back-intellance-2#undefined

- Blurred vision
- Dry eyes
- Swelling of the eye tissue
- Eye pain
- Itchy eyes

- Inflammation of the cornea
- Sensitivity to light
- Watery eyes
- Feeling like something is in your eye

Other common side effects include tiredness and lack of energy

5 October

2.56 pm   Jack's eyes better. He can see more, and we have a range of new drops, which help a lot. No headaches, etc., which is unusual – maybe this shit is working!! Saw the oncologist today and bloods are good so treatment #3 will be tomorrow. MRI in a couple of weeks but I am less concerned about that at this time as he has none of the symptoms that would suggest we should be worried. I don't hope this is a cure as we know from everything we have read it is not but it provides time for other treatments to be developed and available. That said if you do a Google on ABT414, it is one of the most promising new treatments for GBM with high levels of EGFR expression. If we get at least another 6 months (dare I hope … 12??) there is a lot happening in this space and a lot of it is going on in Melbourne at the Olivia Newton-John Research Centre.

Jack's genome sequencing has been comprehensively mapped   3.01 pm by Garvan and while there is nothing there that it feels it can target specifically, as these new therapies are rolled out they are back checked against the database, so Jack might be a candidate for a targeted (yet to be approved) therapy in the future. Just have to keep him alive till then (and that is our job!!).

Re-reading this observation now reminds me of our mantra that was premised on the notion that we cannot beat this devil, but if we can buy time then the next best thing will come along and buy us more time, etc. We also thought where the tumour was located (and largely removed in two operations), that if necessary, Jack might be prepared for further surgery to debulk the mass and again give us more time. But Jack vacillated on that point and said very loudly and passionately after his first operation that he would never do that again. However, within six months he did, although I wasn't sure if he would volunteer for round 3. This was academic anyway and, as it turned out, irrelevant as the new tumour went where a scalpel could not reach it and where it could grow without fear of interruption.

13 October   Jack having problems with his eyes – dry eyes, sore eyes, sensitive to light, very tired eyes. All related to the treatment but he is not having a good time. It makes him irritable and even quieter than usual. Other than that, there are no other "tumour" like symptoms, which is clearly a positive

21 October   JACK UPDATE. Blurry eyes are the big issue but everything else is good. Blood is normal, and an EEG also was normal (neurologist suspected some possible minor seizure activity but that completely ruled out). Have MRI on 31 October and that will guide us on what to do next: change course, pullback on frequency of current medication (ABT414) if all the signs are good or panic stations. The latter I am not a believer in as Jack has no typical tumour symptoms and, other than his eyes, he is feeling very good. I have been dreadfully wrong before but every minor symptom discussed yesterday was sheeted back to the drug and as the oncologist said, "ironically it probably means that the treatment is doing what it supposed to do".

22 October   He has just gone for a walk. Almost bolted out the door. Sure-footed and resolute. Eyes wavering however – from very clear (20/20) to blurred again. I am going to Adelaide this coming week for three days (official open of our new "spat" [baby oyster]) facility). Wasn't going initially as thought might be an issue with Jack but very comfortable at the moment that he is doing well.

OCTOBER NOTES

Dianne contacted Oncology to discuss his eyes and whether there were other treatments we could use to reduce the discomfort. Jack was referred immediately to the RHH Ophthalmology for an eye exam. Mixed results. His peripheral fields had improved especially on the right side. Eye test proved he had BETTER than 20/20 vision. However, there was dryness in his eyes, for which drops were prescribed. This didn't really help though and we arranged a follow-up appointment for two weeks (16 October) to check on progress.

Jack saw the Neurologist on 2 October. This appointment was to determine if Okay to drive, however the discussion morphed into more about his seizure medications and whether this needed to be increased due to presence of the new tumour. Dr Aldous requested an EEG (31 October) to ascertain if there is minor seizure activity causing some of his memory, vision issues. She also prescribed 2mg Melatonin to help with Jack's sleeplessness. He took it that night and it worked fabulously.

Jack saw Oncologist on 3 October for review of his bloods prior to infusion. Platelets had improved slightly to 86, so he was confident to proceed with full dose of ABT414. Eye health is still a concern, so additional measures of cold packs and Visine drops were added.

Friday 4 October was Jack's third infusion of ABT414. All went well, no side effects, except tiredness and eye dryness two days later.

On Tuesday 10 October Jack was very tired, and his eyes were particularly irritated. However, his sleeplessness has disappeared since taking only one 2mg dose of Melatonin on 2 October. Waking up is the problem now!

EEG on 12 October showed no seizure activity; everything "normal".

Ophthalmology on 16 October confirmed cornea toxicity from ABT 414. Prescribed 1% Dex 4x per day. This had immediate positive impact. Most blurry vision went within a day. Dropped back to 3x per day when vision stabilized. Hourly lubricant drops, and evening gel continued. Eyelids still very heavy and remains a huge problem.

NOVEMBER

3 November   Just left Jack. He is having another treatment of ABT414 this afternoon. News not great I am sorry to report. I guess I expected a miracle and the news was sobering. There appeared to be some modest tumour enhancement (so rather than shrinking it appeared to have grown). But only by a very small amount and the fact that it is not associated with increased brain swelling the oncologists aren't convinced it is all bad and maybe the ABT414 is working but slowly. We decided to stay the course with some additional chemo drugs added to the mix. Next MRI is 7 weeks unless we have reason to request one urgently. Jack very disappointed but hasn't wavered from his commitment to beat this sucker. We talked again about him possibly not having much time and he accepts that. I don't and never will.

Although we had many conversations about his mortality he reiterated, in most cases, his unwavering commitment to beat "this". And that stimulated me and I would say then, Mum and I will fight with you and together we will find a solution, I just need more time. But there were other times when he was more despondent (more in his mannerisms as he was a boy of few words) and you sensed his frustration and despair. That would just spur me on more and I would find something and then go to his room with a smile on my face and say something like, "guess who I have just been talking to and guess what they said ?" etc. There were also times when I said these things and then I would just burst into tears and we would switch roles between father and son – he would smile, walk towards me and hug me. Those were the moments I just felt so utterly useless.

If it wasn't doing anything Jack would be dead as the tumour was growing very quickly at the time we started on the ABT414. On the other side, it may have just brought us time, but the outcome is the same.

11 November

But on a sour note, Jack not good. Bad headache led to vomiting and had to call an ambulance last night. Spent night in hospital. Di with him now but we are out of options. Nothing left in the kitchen sink. Don't want to lose him but we hate seeing him like this, hate it.

Jack and Di home. Scan showed swelling around tumour as expected but unsure of cause – new medication or tumour growth. Consensus was new medication and supporting that was the fact his headache peaked and was easing before any medication was administered. The last time this happened was late December last year and showed massive tumour growth and prognosis that he had very little time left. I always want to see the positive side but have miss footed so many times I stopped believing in my own spin. So hope it is the temozolomide that caused the problem and not tumour growth. We have upped his dexamethasone dosage to control the swelling and hopefully it makes a difference.

He is pretty good although obviously very tired. Had a good chat on the way home like nothing had happened.

One thing for sure I am really looking forward to his 21st party on 25 November!

12 November

How is Jack?

11.56 am

Very good actually. On Friday night I wrote him off – deja vu from that horrible December last year. But he is very good. Headaches started after he finished the temozolomide and maybe there is an association,

12.01 pm

but three days of building headaches threw me. I was very messed up as I watched the ambulance drive away. I might be wrong but have my suspicions.

We booked a trip to Sydney. Di not coming now but Matthew, Jack and Chris will be with me. At least at this stage it is still on. It takes a lot to get Dianne back to Sydney and she can use the break.

I have been in correspondence with Professor Hui Gan (Olivia Newton-John Cancer Research Institute) regarding Keytruda, ABT414 and clinical trials. He has been very forthcoming and believes that ABT414 is the best option for Jack at the moment (although this is an opinion without the benefit of reviewing Jack's medical notes) but it is one I strongly support (given the reading and research I have done). The data on Keytruda did not support use in treating GBM at this stage, although there were a number of clinical trials he noted that might be of some interest. A couple were Stage 1 trials so outcome and efficacy completely unknown and untested.

17 November Jack is relatively good. Had a good meeting with the oncologist today and another infusion of ABT414. She appears to be happy with progress. Eyes are an ongoing issue (fixable though when he is off the drug). Don't think he is in great spirits to go out tonight but tomorrow may be different altogether. He has a very lonely existence at the moment (which is unavoidable) although he hides his frustrations well. Just wish sometimes he would scream and start throwing stuff around and saying "why the f**k me!!" but that just ain't Jack's style. He is more 'suck it up princess'.

Looking back on this note I made in November last year, I puzzle why he is proud of the fact that he hasn't cried over his predicament as neither Dianne nor I taught him that. Being a rock and resilient in the face of death gives him strength however, as he hates showing any weakness and, as his brothers have always held him up on a pedestal, I fear that he wants that status to remain unchallenged. Crying or showing emotion would compromise his perception of himself (and in the eyes of others), as this highly competent and confident young man – which I can take if he wasn't dying, but he refuses to concede his situation has irreversibly changed – and for the worse – and everybody sees that.

But as the cycle started to reach its inevitable and horrible conclusion, after Christmas 2017, his vulnerabilities were unavoidably transparent and eventually he stopped caring, as he was no longer in control.

He is OK. Mild headaches daily but also recede to nothing. We are staying on the ABT414 as don't have an option other than maybe Garvan. But the double immunotherapy drugs can also be quite potent. New nurse on day cancer unit from Brisbane tended Jack on Friday and she was involved in ABT trials in Brisbane. Dianne was with him and it gave her some hope, and she became quite animated as she told (and retold) the story.

20 November

Keeping eye open for trials but advice from Hui, my own research and this nurse, suggest the longer we stay the course, the better the possible outcome. Five years ago, Jack would not have been with us as all standard treatments ineffective.

Jack turned 21 today. Wow. How did we get here? Dianne and I had hired the upstairs bar at Jack Greene for the night and invited around 30 of his friends. But typically, Jack, never spend a cent guy, got angry with me when I told him the

25 November

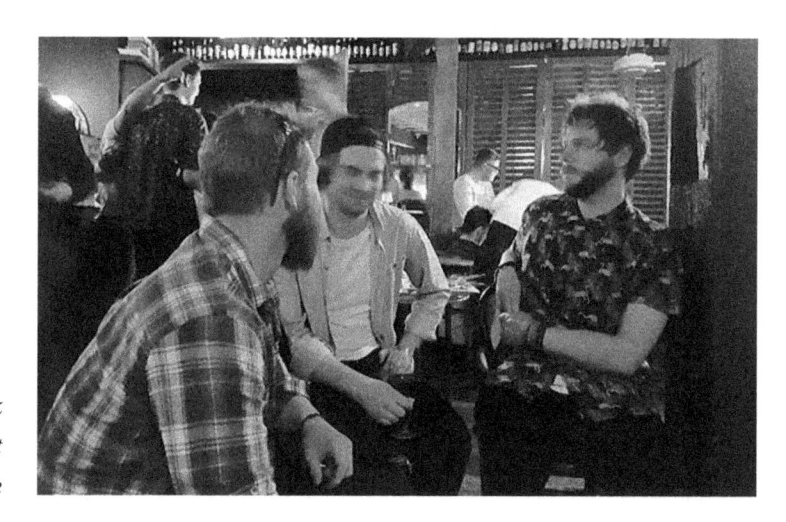

Stefan, Jack and Adrian at Jack Greene

cost would be around \$4,000. He couldn't believe I would spend \$4,000 for his birthday and thought it was so over the top. I said \$1M would be cheap if it made a difference.

I was preparing to make a short speech but wasn't sure how I would hold it together and I let the moment pass. But he was engaged all evening and most of his close friends had few illusions that this could be his last birthday.

Stefan and Adrian stayed with him most of the night just in case there were any issues. And as far as drinking is concerned with the meds he was on and at the same time facing certain death, if the alcohol killed him it would be a kinder and gentler death than getting his brain crushed by an ever-expanding melon that had nowhere else to go. This may seem overly cynical and fatalistic but he had so much taken from him and he wanted to enjoy a couple of whiskies, well fuck it, enjoy a couple of whiskies.

28 November
7.13 pm

Jack received the whisky today and asked me to thank everyone. His eyes are playing havoc and it is messing with his mind. He is not sure who he thanked although thought it was Rosie? Very confused and increasingly frustrated. He said it will be a while b4 he gets around to drinking it and we agreed to share it when this is all over.

We had a frank discussion tonight and I told him there is nothing else we can recommend and even if there were, most of these treatments are embryonic and efficacy unknown. For the moment I said we don't have any immediate options. 7.16 pm

https://en.m.wikipedia.org/wiki/Matt_Price (2007 – diagnosed in October, dead in November). 7.32 pm

As I review my dialogue with my family in this post, Jack now 16 months post diagnosis, I recall he was confused and frustrated at times but, other than arguments with Dianne (she is very black and white) and arguments with his brothers (someone didn't replace a toilet roll or the bathroom handtowel; handing him two tissues when he only asked for one, all being issues that got under his skin) he seemed relatively composed and content. But there were those throw away lines like I know I don't have much time; nothing is working is it? That exposed a more fundamental undercurrent and foreboding that maybe, just maybe, Daddy isn't going to do the impossible. And I would compound my own doubts by finding references to people that faced (and lost) a similar fate, like Matt Price. This also became a constant (and macabre) theme for me and that was rediscovering the history of people that died prematurely (or were suffering) from the same disease that was killing Jack – GBM – and that which in a normal life for me would remain undiscovered: Senator Edward Kennedy; Beau, the son of former US Vice President Joe Biden; Senator John McCain; Matt Price; John Trivett (who I worked for in the 1970s while at Uni); Rona Newton-John (sister of Olivia); George Gershwin; Patrick Cargill, Andrew Olle and the list goes on and on and on. I would read these stories and determine the amount of time they survived from diagnosis and compare that to where Jack was post diagnosis – is he ahead or behind?

DECEMBER

2 December   Text KF ▸ JF

Sleep well my son. You are never alone. Your door is closed, and I walk past it so many times during the day and all I want to do is walk in there and hold you.

You are the bravest person I know: never complain, never give up. I love you so much it hurts.

I can't trade places with you but if I could I would take your place in the blink of an eye.

I love you with every breath I have and hate what you are going through. Hate it and I will never give up trying to find an answer.

Goodnight my beautiful, beautiful son.

10 December   Jack was 17 months post diagnosis on Friday. A good milestone. However, his processing abilities have deteriorated. Not a good sign given where the tumour sits and could mean tumour growth. Jack worried. He has an MRI tomorrow and Dianne and I are less hopeful. Wish I could be more positive but not feeling it.

13 December   Oncology called and want an early meeting with Jack, tomorrow now at 2 pm. Doesn't sound good.

Dinner at a pub in Battery Point tonight. Chris in Devonport with his squeeze, Ashleigh. Chris also got his licence today. Jack desperate for chicken parmigiana.

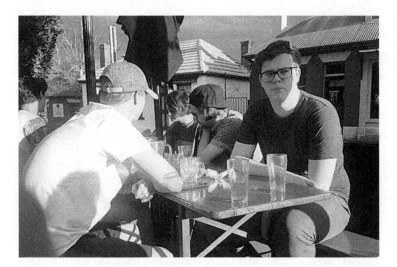

Hugh, back to camera, Jack and Matt

It is all over. Tumour growing and getting into dangerous parts of the brain. Neurosurgeon's view is it is inoperable and even in event he collapses as the tumour grows they would not operate as it is just prolonging the inevitable. Current treatment ceased immediately. There are a few other options which we will consider but neither of the two oncologists are hopeful. Meeting with palliative care nurses in next couple of days/week to discuss end of days. Hard to read Jack's response. Should be the best Christmas however as it will count forever.

John Heath said he thought this will be Jack's last Christmas and I respected his honesty but I like a challenge so I asked if he believed in spontaneous remission and whether he had witnessed it in similar cases? He said no to both. I told him I was "working on it" and both he and Victoria (always there to support Jack) laughed. Gotta stay on song.

He has been given a couple of months, but no one knows, and it could be very sudden.

14 December
3.54 pm

4.00 pm

I remember that meeting as if it was yesterday. Dianne, always more practical than me, knew it and had been making comments regarding the symptoms she was seeing and what she knew to look for as that time drew near. Me? Always in denial but this day, this day, I was gutted and knew I had lost. This day I gave up. This day was an awful day.

22 December   Today I got angry. We have been trying to get a disability support pension approved for Jack and Centrelink has been obfuscating, premised on Jack's investment in Elmside and Fleming Family Trust information for the financial year FY17. The lack of progress over three months and after we had provided Centrelink with all the information requested, pissed me off but more critically, made Jack angry and frustrated. He is dying so we did not need any more anger and frustration. I did my usual dummy spit after Dianne got off the phone again – been sitting on the line for over two hours – and had been told the same bullshit. So I wrote to the Minister (Christian Porter) and pleaded with him to redress the situation:

"However, to add to our frustration, we applied for a disability support pension for Jack who, at that time, we thought there was a (albeit) slim chance he might be with us a little longer. His last MRI (several weeks ago) confirmed that this was wishful thinking. Nonetheless, Centrelink has redefined the word 'delay' and now, three months later, his application is still "under review"!

Maybe it is a conspiracy or I am overly paranoid, but there appears to be a strategy to avoid taking any decision on this application till he is dead!"

Within 24 hours of this post Jack's first payment was processed.

It was a challenging Christmas between the marked deterior- Christmas
ation in Lola's (the family dog) health and Jack's moments of
unadulterated sheer pleasure, mild (and increasing) seizures,
headaches, weariness and near blindness; we experienced
many highs and many lows. I do not generally enjoy Christmas
as the magic I experienced as a child is long gone and the boys
are young men, and Christmas is nothing special for them.
There have been many magic moments when the boys – all six
of them, and at different ages – still believed that Santa Claus
drank some of the milk we left out and ate half the cookie we
left with the milk. But Dianne enjoys Christmas so I try and
get in the spirit.

Chicken parmigiana at the Prince of Wales – Jack's slice
of heaven here on earth.

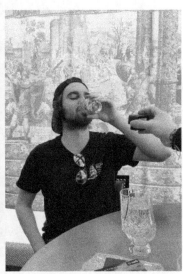

*far left Chicken
parmigiana at
the Prince of
Wales*

*left Glasshouse
(last drinks for a
condemned man)*

Stephanie, Stefan, Jack, Ingrid ("Frenchy") and Adrian

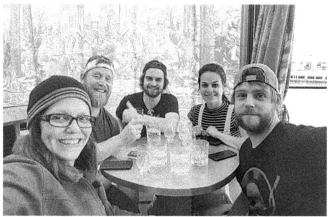

Adrian, Stefan, Chris, Hugh and Matt with Jack seated

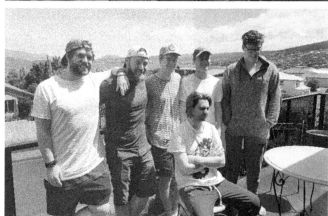

Adrian, Matt, Jack, Hugh, Chris and Stefan

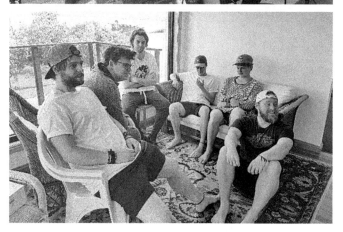

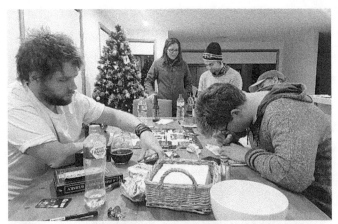

Adrian, Matt, Stephanie and Jack

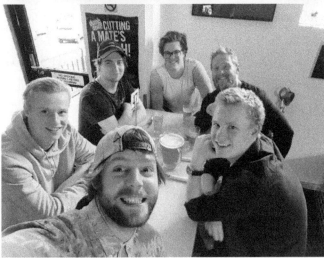

clockwise from front Adrian, Hugh, Jack, Matt, Stefan and Chris at the Prince of Wales Hotel, Battery Point

I have kept the communications on Jack to a minimum as I am still traumatised by what is now the unspeakable reality. Hard to stay positive and can't pretend that nothing outside of a miracle will save him. Disorientation and mild seizures have been increasing although he had some great days/nights with Stefan and Adrian and their partners. His eyes have not improved and are sore and hard to open.

30 December

1.02 pm

To stop (or minimise) the seizures we have increased his anti-seizure medication. He also had his first treatment of the new drug (Avastin), which costs $3,500 each shot, last week. In last couple of days, we have noticed a few things: eye problem unchanged; better cognitive function and no shakes (seizures).

The Avastin is not supposed to change the outcome (that is almost certain short-term death), but improve cognitive function. It has, however, been associated with tumour regression in some cases.

On his eyes, Di took him to the local optometrist and he said his corneas were particularly dry. He already had drops for this problem, but he gave him another medication. I have also done some trading for him in last couple of days and he made $3,500, so that brought a smile to his face.

We set up the Bell Trading account just after he received his terminal illness insurance payout and he asked me to trade for him as he finds it difficult to focus. However, he checked the share prices every day and if anything had fallen he would challenge me and sometimes in his quiet contemplative ("I will leave it then Dad") manner (walk away, downcast eyes), I seemed to always be on the defensive. But if I made money for him I was a hero. And even Dianne would challenge me (and fair enough) as I chose small, eclectic stocks that would run hard or fall precipitously and there was a lot of precipitousness.

1.09 pm   As a footnote, three of our neighbours got together and gave us a large hamper just prior to Christmas. They are feeling it too. And Katrina dropped off a big pack of her special homemade biscuits last night. She is very sweet. Left it outside the door around 9 pm and then sent me a text. So we sent Matt out and left a big bottle of champagne outside her door and I sent her a text.

DECEMBER NOTES

Oncology RHH 1 December – next infusion of ABT414 with TMZ. Added Acetazolamide pill to help with Jack's minor headaches, with the view to reducing the dexamethasone.

He had an ophthalmology appointment on 5 December – confirmed eyes were extremely dry but structure all OK. Continue with hourly BionTears best. Said OK to not take dexamethasone drops except with ABT414 protocol.

Sydney trip for 3 days, left Hobart on 6 December. Oncologist increased dexamethasone to 4mg to fly. No problems during trip other than general tiredness and one small headache.

Bloods taken to check all OK with new Acetazolamide pill on 8 December. Also Stefan's birthday, 32.

calendar 2018

1 January JACK CAME UP THE STAIRS FROM HIS BEDROOM AT around 8.30 in the morning and with a smile that I hadn't seen (it seemed) like forever! He just seemed to be in good spirits. I didn't ask why, just enjoyed the moment.

Dianne started to administer the cannabis oil that we received from a friend in Sydney. The instructions were about a third of a grain of rice, three times a day for several days and then increase the strength. We are not sure how it will react with his current medications and there is no one we can talk to given we are self-administering and the drug's legal status is unknown. There are many variants of cannabis oil and this one is the same one that has been recommended by Rick Simpson (he claims it cured his cancer!).

And there are some good stories online of the cancer fighting benefits of cannabis oil and, at this late stage of the game, what do we have to lose? Jack has a death sentence and all the conventional advice has failed to shift the momentum away from certain death. The words of Ben Williams resonate loudly in our ears and that is, you are on your own and the patient has a death sentence so you can't make it any worse. Experiment and do not only be led by traditional clinical advice as no one has the answer: GBM kills.

Stefan, Stephanie, Jack and I went to the Taste of Tasmania in the afternoon. Dianne drove us in and we had a couple of beers, some barbecued eel and Jack also had some cider. He was in good spirits but admitted later that he felt a little "spacey" (which we put down, rightly or wrongly, to the cannabis oil). He went to bed at around 9.30 as he was very tired but got up at 12.30 am and I gave him a Melatonin tablet.

I got up about 8.30 and found Dianne with Jack in the lounge room. Dianne said that Jack was feeling a little spacey so decided to hold back on the cannabis oil and try and find someone that can give us some advice re the potential complications.

2 January

Jack seemed a little more lost than normal and his eyes are a constant frustration – sometimes semi-clear, other times blurred. He also remarked later in the evening that he felt his "processing" was worse today than it had been in recent days. I put that (quietly) down to the tumour (and quietly hoped I wasn't right).

He was really a lost sheep today. Wandering around the house searching for what I don't know. Just broke my heart.

The boys tried to engage him in a game, but he said that his eyes weren't good. I later went down to see him and asked him how he really was feeling and what was on his mind. He said he thought it was time that he told his friends (through Facebook) what was really going on and that his time may not be long. He had been thinking and writing all day about what he wanted to say and had his Mum help with the words. He also wanted a "sad" photograph of himself to go with the post to reflect the solemnness of the occasion but I said he should have a happy photo that reflected hope because we are still in there fighting. He said he would think about it.

Later, around 10 pm, I was moving ham from one container to another and Jack came up the stairs. "You pig!" he said, with a huge grin on his face. "Too late for you to be pigging out Dad!". I immediately went on the defensive and told him I was only repackaging it and he gave me a smirk, then turned around and went back downstairs.

3 January   Jack seemed fine in the morning except, of course, his eyes. He had an appointment with his oncology nurse at the Royal to talk about how he was going.

Jack keeps his cards too close to his chest and doesn't want to burden anyone with his problems. Thinks this is being tough; a man. And in hindsight, Jack is a lot like me (and I know without even looking at Dianne that she would be nodding vigorously!) and as much I declare I am honest and open, I keep a lot of my musings, frustrations and fears to myself. Think I am the archetypal Australian male but have always encouraged my children to hug (something my father never did) and openly discuss issues. Do what I say and not what I do, but Jack clearly saw through that and mirrored my (sometimes) controlled emotions. And Dianne would say: "He is so like you!". With Dianne on the other hand, you knew exactly what she was thinking and you never had to second guess whether she was angry or happy. Her laughter would fill the house and her anger would raise the roof: black and white; but with Jack and I there is a lot of grey.

Later that day he saw the ophthalmologist to check on his eyes. The ophthalmologist said that it is possible the damage to his corneas, caused by the ABT414, may be permanent. Since Jack has been home Dianne has been putting drops in his eyes every hour.

He ate a small dinner as he wasn't hungry (had a late lunch) and played Cluedo with Matt, Chris and Hugh.

4 January
Wellness 7/10

I was up stretching in the morning before going to the gym (on the ground floor of our house), when I heard Jack's door open and the bathroom door close. It was 6.35 and I knew he would be up early to watch the Arsenal/Chelsea match. Arsenal drew first blood and his smile lit up the room. However, it soon soured as the visitors got one back and then scored again. It finished two-all. Jack swore quietly and left the room. A different boy now, but once he would be so agitated by any Arsenal loss he was like a bear with a sore head all day.

Had a reasonable day but eyes were endlessly sore and "tired". We put eye drops in his eyes every hour.

He went to bed around 10.30 pm, saying he wasn't tired but couldn't see much because of his eyes. I went to bed at 12 but heard him moving around at about 4.00 am.

5 January
Wellness 7/10

I went upstairs to investigate and he said that his knees were aching. I got a towel and two ice packs and put them on his knees and gave him two Nurofen. He said he would be fine and I left him, returning 45 minutes later. He said he was feeling better and went to bed.

He came upstairs around 8.30 am and said that he had (finally) a reasonable sleep.

Dianne investigated the knee issue and said it was a common side effect of the Avastin and we started on a course of turmeric (powder mixed in water or juice) to relieve the swelling (as had been commented on by an Avastin patient that it had stopped all joint pain).

Chatted to him at 11.34 am and he seemed in good spirits. Earlier he had told Dianne that his eyes were "better" today. And he said to me around midday that his "processing" had improved.

He went to bed around 10 pm but came back upstairs about an hour later and said his knees were hurting. We gave him ice packs plus some Panadol and Nurofen. He went back to bed and we didn't hear him get up till the morning.

6 January
Wellness 8/10

He was up around 8 am and said that it took him some time to get to sleep but when he did he said his knees were fine, no pain. He sounds and looks good. Very normal.

He commented early afternoon that his eyes had improved and he felt that his comprehension had also improved.

Overall a good day. He went to a 21st birthday party in the evening and one of his mates said around 11 pm that he was fine.

7 January
Wellness 7/10

He came home around 2 am and woke me. I was asleep on the couch (too many whiskies!). He looked good, comfortable and was smiling. Said his knees were fine but his ankles were hurting a bit. Also said that he had only three beers and was totally sober. I gave him some Nurofen and told him to wiggle his ankles which he did and said that it helped. He put ice on his ankles and then later went to bed.

He woke and came upstairs around 8 am, complaining of ankle and knee pain. Dianne put some ice on his ankles and knees. But besides this, he was in great spirits all day. He spent the most part of the day in the lounge room where he now prefers to be rather than in his room with his door closed.

Minimal discomfort in the evening and Dianne, Jack and I sat down and watched a movie.

A significant day in many ways. Firstly, it was the anniversary of 18 months post Jack's diagnosis – a monumental milestone. Equally importantly and sadly, it was the day we put Lola down. She had cancer which resulted in a large growth on her back. She was also old (12 in August) and had great difficulty lifting her body and walking. It was an emotionally stormy day and all four boys, Dianne and I were there when she closed her eyes for the last time. It was one of the very few times I have seen Jack cry.

8 January
Wellness 8/10

Jack had a good day and didn't need to get up in the night for joint pain. However, he had some modest joint discomfort. Aside from the stress of Lola's last day, Jack was in good spirits and there were no issues.

Jack was not up during the night but arose around 8 am and said he had some very minor (1 or 2 out of 10) joint pain. We understood that on Wednesday Jack was having his next infusion of Avastin but that (and as yet to get confirmation) has been moved to the following week. Our understanding of dosage and that of the pharmacist (and as advised by Jack's oncologist) were different: we understood 1,000 ml every two weeks or 1,500 ml every three weeks. However, it would appear that this was to be 1,000 ml every three weeks.

9 January
Wellness 8/10

Day was uneventful and the boys played Cluedo with Jack in the afternoon. I also came across an article on an

18-year-old girl who was (coincidentally) also diagnosed with terminal brain cancer 18 months ago:
https://www.9news.com.au/national/2018/01/09/13/32/victorian-teenager-suffering-rare-brain-cancer-dealt-another-blow.

I read the article out to Jack but he seemed little interested and walked away. I meant to ask him how he felt about that story later but didn't.

In the evening we went to Blue Eye for dinner where Jack had two glasses of red wine. He commented (good heartedly) that he was the "dumbest person at the table". Dianne quickly reminded him that he was probably the brightest academically but his 'brilliance' was being suffocated by the tumour on his brain.

The boys wandered off around Salamanca to get some dessert while Dianne and I went to a bar. They joined us around 40 minutes later and Chris, Hugh and Jack went home.

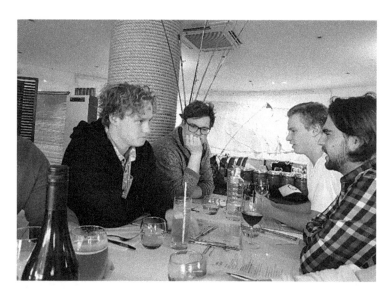

left to right Chris, Matt, Hugh and Jack at Blue Eye

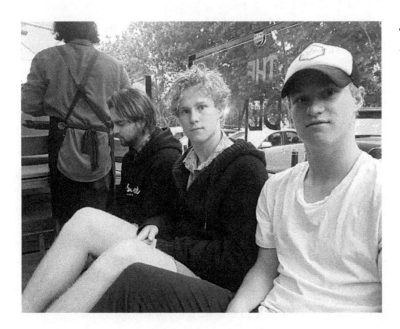

Jack, Chris and Hugh at The Den

When we got home (maybe 10 minutes after them), Jack was sitting quietly by himself in the kitchen sipping on a beer. He had been crying over Lola. We talked about it and told him that it was perfectly normal to cry and no shame in that and in fact it is just a healthy manifestation of deep emotions. He drank a whisky after that, talked for a bit with Stephanie, Stefan, Dianne and I and then went to bed.

A very good day for Jack. There is ongoing joint pain (knees and ankles) but his eyes continue to improve and he is squinting a lot less.

10 January
Wellness 8/10

When I got upstairs at 6 am Jack was in the lounge room and said that his knees were hurting. He had the same issue early evening. Other than that, I do not recall any time recently he has been as happy or laughed as much in a single day!

He went out to the Prince of Wales in the evening with some friends. I drove him in and he talked about Lola and expressed his sympathy for me as I have had three dogs that have died. My first, Whisky, was put down when she collapsed in the backyard. (It was this experience that I had shared with Dianne previously, saying that Lola should be put down here, her home, and surrounded by her family, when she could no longer walk.)

I used WhatsApp to ask his friends how he was and George came back and told me he was fine around 9 pm. He caught an Uber home later and went straight to bed.

I made an appointment with Dr Greg Swartz (Gore Street Medical) for 10 am on 12 January. The practice, and Greg in particular, promote 'alternative' cancer treatments. I am not sure where this will lead but we have nothing to lose.

Jack also has an appointment with his oncologist at 12 tomorrow.

11 January
Wellness 8/10

Another good start. We met with Greg Swartz at 10 am and it was uplifting. He asked Jack a number of questions about his health history and we filled in most of the gaps. I had already sent a missive to him in an email that provided the background as to why we were here. His advice reinforced all that we had read over the previous 19 months regarding supplements, vitamins C and D and the ketogenic diet. It was refreshing as I felt (again and after a long absence) that we had won back some control in fighting this disease. That control has been wrenched from us after his last MRI scan and the very dark and sobering conversation we had with Jack's oncologists in December. Part of that discussion included the inevitable (and I hoped forever avoidable) conversation on palliative care and "next (final) steps".

Greg asked Jack to have a blood test to measure his insulin levels and discussed a range of supplements and vitamins, including adding PSK Trammune (a Japanese mushroom extract), high doses of Melatonin, vitamin D and infusion of vitamin C. He also discussed the ketogenic diet – which we were aware of but to date avoided. It is a high fat diet that has some history in countering epilepsy in epileptics and seizures

Gore St Medical
Integrative Health Centre

Dr Greg Schwarz
MBBS, B.Med. Sci, MSc (Env Mgt)
Nutritional and Enviromental Medicine

started
12/1/18

+ D₃ 25,000 iu/day with food for 10 days, then twice weekly (eg Sat/Sun)

Zinc plus (Metabolic Maintenance) 1 daily with food

Boswellia complex (Mediherb) 1 - 0 - 1
Magnesium citrate 140 mg 1 - 0 - 1

Artesunate injection twice weekly

Ketogenic diet - eg Diet Doctor
Patricia Daly

Melatonin

Intravenous vit C

2 Gore Street   Phone: (03)6224 6717
South Hobart TAS 7004   Fax: (03)86761997
www.gorestreetmedical.com.au

PSK Trammune

in brain cancer patients. It had also shown, in some instances, to attack (and kill) cancer cells. The theory is that cancer cells thrive on sugar and if you cut sugar (direct) and sugar fuels (indirect) you starve the cancer and it cannot grow. As I said, it can also reduce the tumour mass.

As we left the office, I got a call from the office of Christian Porter (Minister for Social Services), apologising for the delay in processing Jack's application for a disability pension. It was a compassionate response to obviously a very sensitive subject as Jack had waited three months for a basic application to be processed. The Minister's adviser confirmed that the "delay" related to the complexity of the application – Fleming Family Trust and Jack's investment in Elmside Whisky – and this had caused the delay. And as I said earlier, within days of my email, Jack's support pension had been fully approved.

I discussed the diet with Dianne later that day and we agreed to consider it.

Jack went out with his friends in the evening and had a good night.

12 January
Wellness 8/10

Uneventful day and Jack again in good spirits. I discussed the ketogenic (or "keto") diet with Jack and he said, 'Dad, whatever it takes. I will do anything and will cut everything out. Just direct me'. I relayed the discussion to Dianne and it was game on. She spent most of Saturday reading about the diet and downloading recipes.

13 January
Wellness 8/10

Another uneventful day. Jack in good spirits and engaged in conversations with Dianne and I for most of the day. He also started walking again – advice that was reinforced in the meeting with his oncologist and earlier with Greg on Friday.

Woke up around 6.45 am and I reminded him that he cannot eat anything or have any beverages (other than water) until he has his blood test. Dianne said later that he woke up feeling a little odd, with a slight headache in the temple region. She put this down to one of the classic symptoms associated with the start of the keto diet – called "keto flu".

14 January

Wellness 8/10

    Good day overall with his good nature and demeanour shining through.

I came in from the gym around 8 am and Dianne had made him an omelette for breakfast. It was a lovely morning and I convinced him to go for a walk.

15 January

Wellness 8/10

    I went to the office and came home around 4 pm. I bought Jack some 78% and 85% cocoa (very dark chocolate) bars which he spotted when I was unpacking the bags.

    "Can I try one", he asked?

    "Yes", I said and gave him several pieces of the 85% cocoa chocolate. He had gone cold turkey on everything that had sugar in it since Sunday and was craving chocolate. High cocoa (70%+) chocolates are OK, in moderation.

    He said it was "good".

    Besides a bad-tempered moment in the early evening when he accused Dianne of misplacing his pills (something Dianne would not have done), it was another uneventful day. Dianne found the pills in the bin so we assumed that Jack had accidentally knocked the container into the bin or absent-mindedly thrown the container away thinking it was empty.

After he vented he sheepishly came back upstairs with a smile on his face and said: "I need structure, as I can't remember shit".

True my son, true.

16 January

Wellness 7/10

Jack spent the morning at the RHH talking in the first instance to Victoria (one-on-one) and having his second infusion of Avastin.

These meetings I later found out were to help Jack deal with the short time he had left and help him say goodbye to the people he loved. Victoria encouraged him to write those beautiful, and final letters, to us all.

I made some "keto coconut bread" (poorly) and cooked up some burgers, which he ate with salad. He liked the bread, but Dianne didn't.

He had a slight nosebleed at the table at dinnertime and a headache developed quickly at the same time. He closed his eyes and seemed uncomfortable. He said the headache came on quickly, on either side of his temple but he was OK.

I went down to see him after he had a shower and he was fine, saying that the headache was only there for a little while but had since gone.

17 January

Wellness 8/10

He was awake early, which appears to be his custom these days. Wakes around 3 am and sometimes goes back to sleep and other times not. I was going for a walk at 7 am and asked him to join me but he smiled and said, he wouldn't.

Dianne later made him scrambled eggs, with a slice of the coconut bread I had made yesterday, smothered in avocado.

I went to the office and Dianne, Jack and I met at Greg Schwartz's surgery at 4. Greg had reviewed Jack's blood test and it showed most key components were within a reasonable range, although his insulin level was unusually high. He said it was critical to get that down as too much insulin results in over-stimulation once a cancer cell has developed, promoting cancer cell growth. He noted that the best way to do that was with strict adherence to the ketogenic diet, which Jack had committed to (and started) on the previous Sunday.

He also recommended twice-weekly Artesunate inject-ions (the first of which he had the following day). Artesunate is used for treating malaria but more recently has been found to be effective against cancer cells. Iron tends to be absorbed at much higher levels in cancer cells than the normal cells and the theory is that this phenomenon causes the acceleration of mutated cells. "Free radicals are formed when iron and oxygen meet and free radicals damage our DNA. This creates a problem with healthy cells; however, in cancer cells it starts mutation and the resistance to therapies grows. Artesunate activates mitochondrial apoptosis as it uses the iron inside the cancer cells against them and causes cell die off." (https://www.anoasisofhealing.com/artesunate/).

He also gave us a prescription to 'high dose' Melatonin, encouraged us to consider a weekly Vitamin C infusion and add boswellia compound to Jack's diet.

When we left the surgery and were standing outside, Dianne lamented that was unfortunate that were speaking to Greg now, rather than a year ago. We had the chance almost a year ago as Greg was recommended to us then, but we didn't follow it up. At the time we both felt strongly that it was an opportunity lost but also in hindsight, we simply didn't know what we were dealing with and what was effective and what was not. We were a normal family with normal family issues and were not built, structured or focused on saving the imminent death of a son from a disease that kills 90% of its hosts in the first 12 months. I mean, where the fuck did that come from?!

We talked about the injection the next day and Jack said, "I don't care, I will do anything that may beat this disease. I will stick to the diet and do everything I have to."

The evening was uneventful, and Jack went to bed at 9.30.

18 January
Wellness 7/10

I was up at 6 am and rang Chris (in the downstairs bedroom) to make sure he was awake for the early (7 am) shift at Mures. He said that Jack had gone for a walk. Even by Jack's standards this was unusual.

When he came home, he said that he was awake (as usual) at 3 am and decided to take an early morning walk. Said he was fine otherwise.

He had his first injection of Artesunate and said it was "painless".

In the evening he was drowsy and a little 'spacey'. Typically, we put this down to all of the usual suspects – tumour, thinking too much (worrying unduly) and the various mix of treatments he is on, including the new (and very strict) diet. It also coincided with the re-introduction of the cannabis oil, which we decided that we will start again. Dianne had given him a higher dose than was recommended for 'starters' and this spacey feeling had followed the second dose.

Jack asked, as he always does when he feels he is not coping well, *is it the cancer causing this issue*? We always say, "it could be" but it could also be the treatments working and upsetting the brain a little.

He went to bed around 10 pm.

19 January
Wellness 7/10

I got up a little later (around 7.30) and when I came upstairs, Dianne was sitting with Jack. Di said Jack's processing wasn't good. He was struggling with words to explain himself. There are moments like these and I fall apart inside and think we are losing him, do we have days, weeks or less?

He later went downstairs and 30 minutes later came back upstairs and said he had a headache. I doubled down on my fears. Dianne gave him two Nurofen and two Panadol.

He had an appointment at the optometrist to review his corneas and the optometrist noted that his corneas had improved markedly, although gave him some different drops/gel/spray for his eyes.

We decided to stop the cannabis oil for the moment as it appears to be the culprit that is causing him all the current cognitive issues (at least that is what we thought). At lunchtime he appeared to be more communicative and engaged.

I related a story to him that Dianne had found on the web regarding Pablo Kelly, 28, from Devon, UK, who was diagnosed with GBM (inoperable) in 2014 and had regressed his tumour by 90% over two years by, he believes, adopting the keto diet and consuming a range of supplements (https://www.dietdoctor.com/low-carb/keto/brain-cancer). Jack was quite chuffed and mentioned it several times during the day with a big smile on his face.

As his short-term memory deteriorated we started writing him notes for when he was out. The two pubs that he used to frequent were Shipwright Arms and Prince of Wales, both in Battery Point. This is the text I sent him on 19 January so that he would know what to ask for when he was at ether venue.

K   At Prince of Wales, whisky selection poor. They have Hellyers Road (slightly peated) and Kilchoman (Islay Scotland), plus usual Irish (Jameson) and cheap American bourbons (Jim Beam; Jack Daniels, Makers Mark, etc.). I would go for the Kilchoman every time but not cheap ($12 a nip). but lovely whisky. Otherwise I would go for the Hellyers.

At Shippies, they had Dalwhinnie (Speyside Scotland), Teeling (Irish) and Hellyers Road. They sometimes have TALISKER, plus usual Irish and American whiskies.

At Shippies I would go Dalwhinnie #1 (lovely whisky); Talisker if they have it (delicious peaty whisky) and Hellyers third. But if you like Irish, Teeling is a good Irish whisky.

I don't mind the occasional Hellyers though.

21 January
Wellness 8/10

Was a good day. Jack engaged and eyesight improved. However, he remarked on several occasions that he was frustrated by his inability to reason and remember basic things. Nevertheless, he was in good spirits and joked with us during the day.

He went out with George Cretin (a very close friend) in the afternoon for a coffee as George was leaving to go overseas for several years. Jack asked me what he could have and I said green tea or black coffee. He later sent me a text with a picture of the beverage menu and said "which one" (he had forgotten that I told him to have a long black with cream):

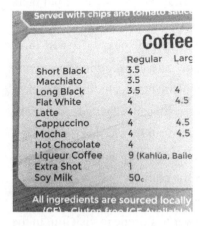

> **J** *Which one?*

K Long black

> **J** *Thanks*

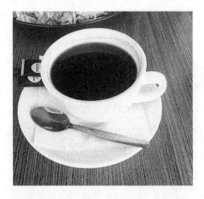

> **J** *Plain black, albeit they made it quite big! Is this correct?*

K Yep perfect.

I made lunch for Jack: half a piece of salmon cooked in butter with salt and pepper, plus a salad and one piece of keto bread with butter.

I made tandoori chicken, keto style, for dinner.

He has had some minor headaches but we have put them down to body adjustments on the new (now one week old) diet. Dianne told me she now believes that the next MRI will show some retracement of the tumour. She is becoming increasing confident that the diet and supplements, including the twice-weekly injections of Artesunate, are a game changer. I hope she is right but, nonetheless, she was usually the more pragmatic and practical of us both and I felt buoyed by her confidence and hoped maybe her intuition was the reality.

In the afternoon I sent George a text wishing him good travels and said I will get Jack over to Europe to visit him in the next 9 months.

Jack went to bed around 11.30.

22 January
Wellness 8/10

I heard Jack moving at around 6 am. When I saw him, he said that he was fine but had (typically) been awake since 3 am. He decided to go for a walk.

Dianne checked his ketones and they were 0.7 (close to 1.0 is good). They were 0.2 several days ago.

I went to the office and got a call from Dianne around 1.45 asking me when I was coming home as Jack was not in a good mood and being rude regarding his "meal plans" and the ingredients he wanted to buy from Woolworths. She was exasperated which is not unusual for Dianne but she usually sorts its out and it is not normal for her to ask for my help in a situation like this. Then again, what is normal now? When I came home around 50 minutes later he was sound asleep and Dianne was out with Matthew. I made some keto bread and later he came upstairs and was very polite.

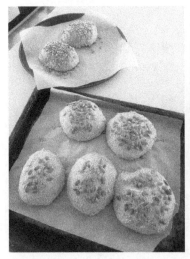 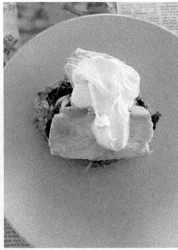

Keto bread rolls and dinner

However, after dinner he wanted to show me a page on alcohol that is recommended on the keto diet. With Jack, he has trouble reading and has trouble comprehending, which when added to his hearing loss, it can be very frustrating having a conversation, particularly if it centres around something written down. Thus, when speaking to him you have to raise your voice and speak a little slower. If you have to read a lot and then talk to him slowly with a raised voice it can be awkward. However, we are used to that but now with his cognitive abilities compromised and his short-term memory almost non-existent, conversations can be exhausting.

Generally, repeat of previous days: Jack in good spirits; totally committed to the diet (no concessions, no compromises, no problems) and engaged.

23-24 January
Wellness 8/10

25 January

Wellness 6/10

Day started normal but, in the evening, Jack said he felt a little weird. Something was going on inside his brain that he could not explain but said it was not normal, although "isn't like a seizure". It is moments like these when all my confidence shatters like a glass wall in an earthquake. He was in the lounge room and we got him to lie down; we put cold face washers on his forehead and Dianne massaged his legs. After 30 minutes he said that he felt incredibly tired and we walked him to bed.

We are never sure how to explain these moments to Jack as we cannot explain them to ourselves! Dianne just said there is like "some movement" which covers a multitude of bases, including tumour growth, cancer cells dying and the adverse effect of the new diet. My fear is that it is the cancer growing as I have always previously looked at these situations as the glass half full (me typically trying to spin it), but now I was becoming more cynical and the glass was always half empty.

Jack woke up well (although he had been having headaches most mornings and coincidentally only since he started the keto diet) and didn't initially remember the episode the night before. However, as we talked it started to come back to him as did the same theme: "Should I be worried the cancer is growing again?".

Every headache or 'odd' feeling he would repeat the same lament, "should I be worried?"

But he had some lunch and I drove him to Battery Point where he spent the day and most of the evening with his friends and having a ball.

K How you doing? 5.55 pm

J *Yeah completely fine. Just put second set of lubricant eye drops In for you. No headaches at all. One of my mates is having a nap now (has been asleep for almost 2 and a half hours now) haha. It's his house.*

Had that same odd feeling after breakfast and a headache that wouldn't dissipate. Dianne took his blood readings and surprised that even though strictly on the ketogenic diet, his ketone count had fallen to 0.5 (0.8 two days ago).

Di decided (and with Jack's agreement) that he should fast (part of the keto diet, so we weren't flying blind). He asked for a coffee around 1 pm and said that he was "perfectly fine" but feeling a little tired.

He went to bed at 11 pm.

29 January

Wellness 4/10

I was up early to exercise and Di and Jack woke up early also. Jack decided to go for a walk and I left a little later and caught up with him. At the 15-minute mark he turned around and started to walk back along the river track and I kept going on my normal walk. If he kept going, he should have been at least 5 minutes in front of me but he came in 2 minutes after me. He said that he also went for a short run but his headache worsened so he sat down and rested before continuing home.

I had breakfast and Dianne cooked Jack's breakfast while I had a shower and dressed ready to go to the office.

When I came back upstairs 15 minutes later to say goodbye, Jack was lying down across three chairs and Dianne was massaging his head. She indicated to me that his head wasn't good. He was certainly not with it although it did not have all the classic signs of a seizure, such as shaking and unconsciousness.

I let my colleagues know I wasn't coming into the office and we walked Jack down to his bed and got him to lie down. He was stressed that he couldn't remember anything (including going for a walk and a run) and was convinced his tumour was growing and causing these problems. He eventually went to sleep.

Dianne and I had agreed some time ago that the lawn needed top dressing and a truck had dumped a huge pile of top soil in our driveway that morning. We left Jack and went out into the garden to barrow and spread the top soil.

After about an hour I went back inside to check on Jack and he was sitting up and dressed in warmer clothes. He was crying and visibly very distressed. "I can't remember anything," he cried. "When was my last MRI? Is this because of the tumour?" Jack was scared. Dianne had opined earlier (and even later) that it was the new meds and/or the diet. I thought of a more darker reason. My fear – and I expressed this to Dianne and within earshot of Hugh, as I wanted to put everyone on notice – that his time could be short and he knows that. We need to have a reality check and it may just be meds and diet or it may just be what we all fear the most.

Jack asked the same questions several times: what day was it; did he go for a walk in the morning; what had happened; did he eat breakfast … over and over and over again … is it the cancer back?, when was my last MRI? Jack was distressed and inconsolable.

As the day progressed he settled and surprised himself as he started to remember the earlier events of the day and with each recollection, he smiled and nodded to himself.

There was no recurrence although having a conversation with him was becoming more difficult as he remembers very little.

He was fine over dinner and came up at 7.30 for a small glass of wine and a game with Chris and Hugh. During the game he became quite animated and totally immersed himself in the game. It was great to hear him laugh.

He went to bed at 9.30.

30 January
Wellness 8/10

He woke around 7 am and sent Dianne a text saying that we needn't be so quiet around his room as he was awake. I went down to see him and he was in good spirits but said that he hadn't slept well and showed me screen shots of his home screen on his mobile taken each time he had awoken. He was thinking of going for a walk but in the night his knees were sore so he thought he would wait till there was less pain. However, he then said that his knees were a lot better now.

He worries and focuses on things that don't matter, like getting reimbursed by the government for medical expenses; why the bottle of antiseptic is not in his room (this is a line repeated daily and he can get quite angry); Hugh using his comb ...

In the afternoon, the twins and Matt took him to Eastlands, for shopping and later bowling. They said he was great and really enjoyed himself. And in the second game when he started to get the hang of it (yes, he had forgotten the game!) he nearly won!!

He was in good spirits when he came home and no issues before he went to bed.

That said, there is an ongoing theme of constant, albeit slight headaches (1, 2 and occasionally 3 out of 10), as well as something "not feeling right" in his head. And he talks a lot which is the complete opposite of Jack's (previously) normal solitary demeanour. He did not engage in conversation unless pressed and gave very little away of his private life (a closed book). Now he never shuts up, although the conversation is repetitive: regarding his absolute commitment to the diet; his total dedication to anything he should take or do that will help him beat the cancer; his temperance willpower; will never feel any criticism of Dianne and I if, ultimately, we fail and he succumbs to the disease; his constant fear that every headache or "weird" feeling in his head is the cancer winning (and him losing) etc.

His need for conversation I think stems from the fact that he feels death is close and senses his vulnerability. It is fear of being alone; of dying alone. But it can be comical sometimes also as he will constantly interrupt Dianne and

I to talk about trivial things. Tonight, for instance, we were watching a movie and he came into the lounge room about five times in 40 minutes and each time as he entered he signalled that we should stop the movie as he had something to say. Well he didn't say much other than I just want to thank you guys for all that you are doing, the diet is amazing etc.

Jack had his third Artesunate injection today at 10 am, at Gore Street Medical. Has had a slight headache most of the day, which we have been treating with Panadol and Nurofen. He has also had a feeling of dizziness and a little nausea.

31 January
Wellness 7/10

However, he enjoyed (and remembered!) a video I showed him taken over Christmas when he was out with Stefan, Adrian, Ingrid and Stephanie. I think it was T42 and after they had come back from a trip to Mona. He laughed, as he was quite vocal and animated in the video and obviously in good spirits. He also asked the date of when he was first diagnosed with GBM (8 July 2016) and then calculated (correctly) that on 8 February 2018 he would be 19 months post diagnosis, a big milestone for someone who was given just 12 months on that fateful, cold, wet afternoon in July 2016.

He lay down later in the afternoon as his head was throbbing and even though he said later that he did not sleep, he said he felt much better.

Dianne (with Hugh driving and Matthew) drove him to the Prince of Wales in Battery Point where he was meeting friends. Several texts in the night confirmed he was feeling good and enjoying himself.

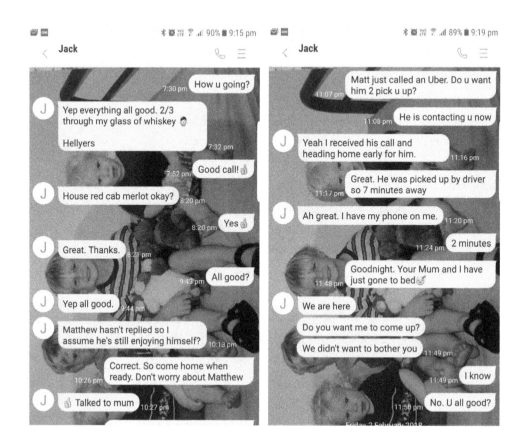

He rang Dianne at 10.20 pm and said he was fine and was about to catch an Uber home. He had had two drinks – one Hellyers Road whisky and one house red and a lot of water.

Matt later picked him up in an Uber and they both came home together. He came in to see us and was in good spirits.

FEBRUARY

1 February

Wellness 5/10

Jack in reasonable mood in the morning but frustrated by constant headaches and 'brain freezes'. His comprehension and processing has shown no noticeable improvement since we started the Avastin or other non-classical treatments, including the keto diet.

Dianne has been concerned all day that his 'fuzziness' may be related to low blood sugars as his readings move around a lot and she doesn't know what they mean. I contacted Gore Street Medical and asked for Greg to phone Dianne back to discuss. He did and made an appointment for 4.30 on 2 February.

I spoke to him tonight as he asks why is he feeling like this – is it the diet, the new treatments or the cancer? This topic is raised several times every day and it has the same answer: we do not know; it could be all of the above. He is feeling vulnerable and knows in his own mind that it is the cancer and his time is short. He said lately he has "been feeling like shit".

I am persuaded to believe him (but believe me, I resist that thought as much as I accept it). He said that his friends keep asking him how much time he has left and he said he tells them maybe a month. He might be right and even optimistic the way I am seeing it.

I get up early four mornings a week and work out in our home gym three mornings a week (walking on the fourth morning). Those times when I am alone I cry a lot. I don't plan it, it just happens.

I think if we could find a way for him to get at least one decent night's sleep, it would make a huge difference as he wakes 2, 3 times a night and struggles to get back to sleep.

He went to bed at 10 pm. It is now 10.30 and I am going to do the same.

Jack had a good sleep and was chuffed that he had only woken twice in the night (!), although in both instances he had quickly gone back to sleep. He was very chatty about it.

However, before breakfast he became nauseous and that lasted for at least 90 minutes.

His consulting nurse rang up and advised that his blood test results were excellent and there was nothing unusual. I came home at 12.30 to play tag with Dianne who was going out with Hugh. He was fine in the afternoon and noted that he always felt better in the afternoon. He also talked about going out with his friends and I said don't ask us, ask yourself and if you feel up to it, then go!

We met with Greg Schwartz in the afternoon. Greg said his blood results were exceptionally good and unusual given that he would have expected some deterioration with the advanced stage of Jack's cancer.

He suggested the nausea could be the result of several things, including negative signals from the brain manifesting in the stomach. He confirmed that we were doing everything right but suggested we add more salt to his diet and that he exercises daily and gets some more sun.

Di, Jack and Matthew played Hop and Pop. It is a simple board game played with dice and the number you roll determines where you can move on the board. It is as complex as Snakes and Ladders but can be a bit of fun and there are tactics so we usually had a laugh. Dianne usually laughs harder and longer than anyone and she really gets into the game but tonight Jack seemed to have more fun that anyone.

When I got up around 8 am Di said that Jack had gone back to bed after getting up early and going for an hour's walk. He was fine.

He sent me a text at 9.30 and asked me to come to his room. He had a big smile on his face and said that he had a good sleep after the walk and was ready for breakfast, as he needed to take his medications.

He has been in great spirits all day. He had a short nap after lunch and then, as per the doctor's instructions, sun-baked for an hour, which he said made him feel really good.

He went out in the evening with friends and didn't get home till after 2 am.

4 February
Wellness 8/10

Jack was up early and complained of significant knee pain. Dianne told him to go to bed and sleep, which he did. He came back up around 8.15 and was struggling to walk. We got him to rest on the couch in the lounge room and Dianne put some ice on his knees. At around 9.30 he said the pain had almost disappeared.

It was an exceptional day and he remarked several times that it was a good day. Had a little nausea however after dinner that we are now associating with the MCT oil. He also noted that he had fewer headaches in the last couple of days and thought maybe he was at a turning point? He had these positive comments and thoughts all day, which were a delight to observe. He was also less thirsty which we collectively put down to adding a little salt to his water (the trick that Greg had advised).

He went for an hour's walk in the afternoon, which he enjoyed.

In the evening he played a game of Pop and Hop with Chris, Hugh and Matthew and drank two very small glasses (very slowly) of red wine.

I went down to see him at 9.50 pm to wish him goodnight and he again remarked about his lack of headaches and general wellbeing. I kissed him on the forehead and said 'goodnight' – something I hadn't done since he was a little boy.

5 February

Wellness 8/10

An uneventful day, with Jack in good spirits.

He played Pop and Hop with Chris, Hugh and Ashleigh (Chris' squeeze).

6 February

Wellness 3/10

I was up early to exercise but I heard Jack moving around about 5.20 am. He said he was fine and had no knee pain but couldn't sleep. I suggested he take a walk and he went out for about 40 minutes.

He had another injection of Artesunate and met later with his oncologist. The oncologist remarked how well he was looking and (I think) was pleasantly surprised. Jack more confident that he is improving (rather than declining) and quite chuffed. I think the signs are more positive than negative, but this disease is crafty and just when you think you have a break, it is snatched away again.

At 7.20 pm I suggested he join me on the balcony for a whisky as it was a balmy 22 degrees. He said sure, and went to his bedroom to get his sunglasses. When he came back up something had changed. He looked bemused and said there was something going on in his head. At that point he had almost a complete short-term memory loss and started feeling nauseous.

We finally got him to bed and he slept well.

7 February

Wellness 2/10

Jack entered a loop last night and has been in it all day – no memory, sheer frustration at not remembering, asking the same questions and then copious tears. He spent most of the day at the Royal undertaking tests including an MRI. Dianne is beside herself as she gets frustrated very easily and has the patience of a fly – meaning she has none. Jack is very challenging at the moment and even I, who can be very measured and patient, am feeling increased frustration from repeating the same answers every 10 minutes.

I think the MRI will show tumour progression, which would explain the memory loss due to blockages forming in his brain.

I think his time is short.

Well that was what I thought and then the game changed and that thought was smashed by the phone call we received from Jack's oncologist, around 9.30 pm. The MRI was inconclusive although one part of the tumour had actually shrunk!! The area that controls short-term memory appears, however, to be experiencing oedema, which is causing his current (extreme) memory loss. One conclusion of that is that the tumour cells are dying and causing swelling? Or, the more obvious!?

The results, therefore, were encouraging (Dianne and I were actually jumping out of our skin as she had the call on speaker) and it was recommended he continue with the Avastin and also take some Rivotril to calm him and help him sleep.

We cried tears of joy.

We did that and related the good news from Rosie, which he found difficult to comprehend.

8 February
Wellness 2/10

Jack started to move around at 5.40 am and Dianne went into to see him. He was dressed but disorientated so no change from last night.

Today however is highly significant for another reason – it is Jack's 19th month of survival following his diagnosis on 8 July 2016. This is a major milestone (but he is too distressed and disorientated to understand its significance – at least for now).

The day was a mirror image of the day before, with Jack in tears a lot and struggling to understand why he can't remember anything. The same questions get asked and statements made: when did I have my last MRI; was the news bad; I thought I had died and come back; is Chris and Hugh back at school; is Matthew back at Uni; where are my two brothers (referring to Adrian and Stefan); I remember a recent holiday when we were all away for at least a week etc.

We try and comfort him but the cycle starts again every 15 minutes and we have not seen any sign of improvement. Dianne and I (unfortunately) can become quite exasperated.

His keto reading was fabulous: 1.2!

9 February

Wellness 2/10

No improvement today. Repetition of the last three days.

He went to the Royal for his Avastin infusion at 8.30 am and later, at 5 pm, visited Greg Schwartz in his Gore Street surgery for an Artesunate injection and consultation regarding Jack's memory loss. Greg could not help with the memory loss but reinforced the anti-inflammation benefits of the keto diet.

I picked up Indian for dinner and Jack enjoyed the chicken tikka, a small serving of butter chicken, salad and a small piece of garlic naan (bad on the diet but hard to keep everything from him at this time given all that he has been through and reasonable probability that his time may be short).

Some modest improvement over these two days, but Jack more relaxed and less anxious. Starting to remember that his memory loss is due to swelling and "temporary" and that his recent MRI was "good news".

His demeanour is more relaxed and he jokes with his brothers who also engage him in games in the afternoon and early evening.

He remembers a basic meditation technique and closes his eyes and calms his breathing. He also recalls that this is a technique that I showed him and he tells me that each time he starts the exercise. He also says he remembers that he needs to do this to avoid another panic attack and he has had a few over the last week, which almost resembles a seizure with his body shaking and he looking visibly distressed.

He is like a small child and states many times during the day how he has total faith in Dianne and I to get him through this.

He is crying less although sometimes you look at him and the tears are streaming down his face.

The day started the same although Dianne's exasperation is all too often on show.

Yesterday I bought a jigsaw puzzle, and a couple of games for him. He walks up and down the stairs several times a day between his bedroom and the kitchen and when he passes these items he repeats the same thing – *I am having a little bit of déjà vu as I am sure I have seen these things before*. We indulge him when he adds, *I am freaking out a bit*. And I always say: "Don't freak out, just stay calm and breathe slowly". And he always says, "I will, I will; I do that thing you showed me".

In the last ten minutes, he has been up twice and we went through the same Groundhog Day moment.

Day played out the same.

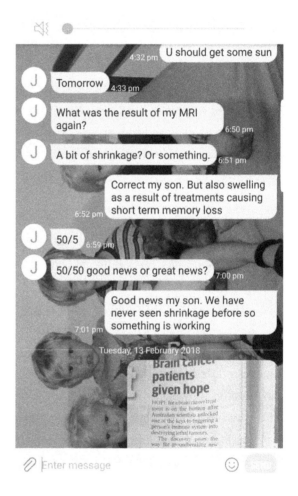

13 February

Wellness 6/10

Jack's demeanour improving and there are moments when his memory shows snippets of improvement. He was up early to watch Tottenham play in the EPL and I asked him how he felt. "Good" he said "and I had a great night's sleep".

At 5 pm he had another appointment with Greg for his Artesunate injection. I came home at 7 pm and he was in good spirits and Dianne said it was an uneventful day. Critically, he is a lot calmer and is now comprehending that this condition is temporary and he has to relax.

Odd day for me as I felt very weak; almost flu-like. It would have been over 10 years ago that I had a similar feeling; very rare for me to ever get ill. Good day to be ill though, as weather was almost cyclonic and the traffic was chaos.

14 February

Wellness 6/10

But Jack in good shape and more comfortable with his severe memory loss. From Wednesday last week, I would say at a pinch that there has been a 5% overall improvement (but I also think other times I am kidding myself).

I have concertinaed these days as they are a mirror image of previous couple of days. The odd headache (but a lot less) and his mood/demeanour has been very pleasant.

15-18 February

Wellness 6/10

We met his oncologist on Friday and she was pleasantly surprised just how good she thought the MRI was and that blew us over, again. We both had read the actual report the night before and it seemed a little more negative than we were led to believe. I have not seen his oncologist this animated in several months and this consultation was different. She was particularly excited about the fact that where there was shrinkage, it was in the Corpus Callosum area of the brain. This area sits between the two sides of the brain and the fear in December was that as that area became invaded, it would stop the blood flow and cause almost instant death. At that time, it was acknowledged his time was short.

Although I am careful not to draw too much from this conversation, as my best hopes have been smashed back in my face too many times previously, so I would be an idiot if I didn't simply add it to the mix and wait for the next day to unfold.

He went out Saturday night and had a ball. Got home around 2 am this morning. Had been texting me all night so I was comfortable he was in good shape and good hands.

He has just gone to bed now and never seems to appreciate just how tired he can get in the evening. We tell him the same thing – he doesn't usually sleep well and of course his body is fighting a life-threatening disease.

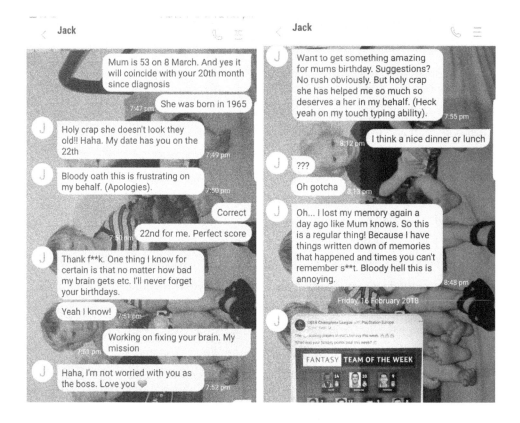

Started out badly – Jack up at 1.30 am with an aching knee – a common complaint and this time we believe it is related to the Avastin. He was in good spirits but uncomfortable. I asked him if he wanted me to get some ice and he said he just taken another Melatonin and was OK.

I got up early and heard him moving around at 7 am. He came out of his bedroom and said that his knees were sore. I wrapped an ice bandage around both knees and Dianne gave him some Nurofen. He recovered quickly.

I rang Dianne late in the afternoon and said I was coming home and how was Jack. She said he had gone for a long walk and worn himself out, although he had a good day. When I came home at 5.45, he looked a little stressed and said, "I feel a little funny in the head. I swear this has happened to me before. I can't remember anything". I said the same thing I had been saying for two weeks – my well-worn mantra: yes, once before but we are working on making it better. He was shivering and said that he was cold, but he was about to have a shower. I put the heaters on in the bathroom and he had a shower.

He later had dinner and then came into the lounge room where Dianne and I were watching the news on TV. "I swear this has happened to me before", he started. Dianne and I looked at each other and then took turns to repeat the ritualistic mantra. However, I sensed something was wrong. I asked him did he remember dinner and he said no. Did you remember having a shower earlier on? He touched his hair and said it was wet but didn't remember having a shower. Did you remember going for a walk today? "No." Up until that moment, he was remembering things he had done at times during the day (snippets) but this was another (complete) clean sheet.

He also said that his headache was not good and said it was a 7/10. Dianne promptly gave him some Nurofen to go with the Panadol she had given him 10 minutes earlier.

But this time, unlike the first time, he didn't panic and sensed that it would be all right, as long as he stayed calm. And stay calm and relaxed (although a "little freaked out") he did. His headache disappeared, and we put him to bed at 9.30.

We believed then that maybe the swelling had become a problem in correlation with the reduction in his dexamethasone medication (recommended by his oncologist on Friday).

20 February
Wellness 6/10

I saw him in the morning when he woke up. Smiling. Said he knew he has some memory loss but it will come back, and he had a good sleep.

I came home around 4 and he was trying to have a nap. He was good and had spent some time in the sun. Later he had dinner and I poured him a small whisky (Japanese – his favourite) and he played several games of Connect Four with Dianne (winning two I recall?) and then played a game of Pop and Hop with Dianne, Matt and myself. He won.

He went to bed and had a great night's sleep.

21 February
Wellness 5/10

He slept well but I didn't see him before I left for the office around 9.15. But Dianne informed me that he was good and didn't have a headache and felt fine.

When I came home Dianne said his head was "funny" for part of the day and he complained again about the "bump" at the back of his head was aching. It was where he had two brain surgeries, but we are (as is the oncologist) unsure why that is hurting. The pain (I understood at the time) was external, not internal.

However, the longer I spent with Jack the more comfortable I became with his wellbeing. He was fine, just constantly annoyed that he had lost his memory and wasn't well enough to go out with his friends this evening. They were meeting at the Prince of Wales.

I ordered Indian and Jack came with me to Bellerive to pick it up. He was bright and chirpy in the car and we talked about his cancer and how he must focus on one thing, and forget everything else, and that is getting better.

Later he played Connect 4 – beat Dianne once and she beat him once and then the three of us played Pop and Hop. I later spent time in his room trying to do some of his jigsaw puzzle that I bought him and we talked some more. He went to bed at 10 pm.

The days have been largely repetitive but Jack in good spirits.

22-25 February
Wellness 3/10

However, there were a couple of events of note, the latter being the most devastating:

- Adrian was down over the weekend, returning to Melbourne on the morning of 26 February. They (as always) bonded well and played chess and a couple of other board games. Jack a lot slower but generally happy and communicative;

- Saturday night he went out to a farewell party at Shippies. I dropped him off at 5.15 pm and he didn't get home till 2.50 am Sunday morning. I was up early on Sunday and he came up to the kitchen around 7 am, with the biggest smile on his face. Had a good sleep (could not have been much!) and had a really good time with his friends;

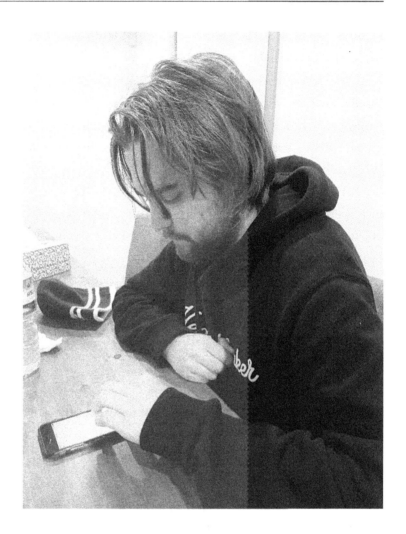

- On Sunday Adrian took Hugh, Matt and Jack to play mini golf and tenpin bowling. Chris was working. When Jack came home he looked lost and said he had lost his memory again. A complete wipe and we start again. He was weeping and, as we have seen in this situation before, he was completely lost.

I heard him get up to go to the toilet at 1.30 am but he went back to bed and closed his door.

This morning started as it always did, "I am so confused … I am sure I have said this to you before, but I have lost my memory …" I reassured him several times that it was all part of his treatment and he should just relax and get better.

Same routine and confusion as the evening before.

Same confusion in the morning. We went to Gore Street Medical for Jack's 10.30 am Artesunate injection. We then had coffee before I walked the last 300 metres to the office.

I didn't notice much change in Jack after I came home at 4.30 and he was again fixated by the fact that Adrian had gone back home and he couldn't remember him leaving. He also cycles through his calendar and asks the same questions, every 20 minutes. I sounded a little irritated the last time he asked and he got quite defensive. So, I said to him you ask the same questions every 20 minutes … and he says, "But Dad, I can't remember!".

I said, "I know but we remember and because you can't, we tell you the same thing but nothing sinks in. So it is useless telling you something that you don't remember" and he said, somewhat frustrated, "then I won't ask!".

I said "Jack, I don't mind you asking but you are not learning anything if you have to repeat the same question every 20 minutes. So how about adding notes in your calendar so when you look at an appointment you know you have asked us that question and the explanation is written down?". He liked that idea.

But subtly, very subtly, I have noticed that he is starting to remember little things. And this just happened tonight. Di said she had noticed the same during the day. But I am not going to jinx this thought with too much analysis but I feel something has changed for the better.

He just came up and said it is "your anniversary on Friday!" And I said yes, 22 years married and 26 years together. I also added "26 years too long" to which he had a good laugh.

28 February - MARCH 4 March Wellness 6/10

I haven't maintained a daily journal as most days are repetitive. Health-wise and ignoring the "memory loss" issue, Jack's health is no less than robust. There are occasional 'slight' headaches but nothing debilitating and he never looks uncomfortable. Telling is the fact that he never wakes up with a headache, which we have been warned (headache in the morning) is not a good sign. He wakes up with a smile on his face and reminds us (again!) that he lost his memory.

We went out to dinner on Friday night – Jack, Matt, Di and I – with a friend and principal shareholder in our whisky company, Peter Camm. It was a good night and Jack, while in good spirits, struggled with conversation with Peter. Dianne and I have never celebrated our wedding anniversary (22 years on Friday) but Peter was keen to catch up and Dianne rarely gets out of the house, particularly for dinner. And Jack refused to go out with his friends and instead insisted on spending the evening with us because it was our "special day".

As I noted before, the bond that Dianne and I had mattered to Jack more than any of the other three boys. It was his rock and I also thought one of the reasons that Jack would never leave home was because our relationship gave him strength and security that he felt (I surmised) he could not experience elsewhere.

Chris and Hugh couldn't make it as they had a football game on.

Jack had both his Avastin infusion and his Artesunate injection on Friday – midday and 4.30 respectively.

This afternoon and tonight, however, he just seems a little more with it and Dianne made the same observation. He doesn't see it and was puzzled when I said that I had noticed some improvement. But it was noticeable. His ketone reading was a massive 1.7 (great news) and his blood sugar reading was around 5 (excellent). His eyes are also getting better daily as he was nearly blind while on ABT414.

Chris has spent some time with Jack over the weekend and took him shopping on both Saturday and today. Jack was very keen to buy Dianne a present for her birthday on Thursday which, coincidentally, is 20 months since diagnosis for Jack. An event I never thought I would see.

He is in his room at the moment watching a movie on his laptop and seems content.

5 March
Wellness 4/10

Slept well and slept in till we woke him at 9.30 am. Seemed fine at the time but very forgetful when I came home and we had several conversations. Nothing staying put for longer than 30 seconds.

I bought home a BBQ chicken and took a drumstick down to Jack in his room. He said he was full but wanted the drumstick. An hour later I asked him if he was hungry and he said "didn't I have dinner?". I said, no but I gave you a chicken drumstick around 5. He said, "Really? I don't remember that". I went to the bathroom and then came back past his room and he was rummaging around in his garbage bin. I said have you lost something and he said he was looking for the drumstick. I said you put the bones in the bin in the kitchen.

I sat down with him after dinner and said you need to make notes. He agreed and then started asking me the same questions and making the same statements regarding his "swelling" and the fact that he can't "remember a fucking thing!". And I say, do you know how many times you have said that and he says, "Said what?".

He was just going down to have a shower but I noticed him on his bed 10 minutes later. I said did you have a shower and he said, "No, do you want me to … didn't I have a shower yesterday?".

Di said he was like that for most of the day.

He came up later to the kitchen while brushing his teeth and handed Dianne his tube of toothpaste and asked her to clean the lid for him. Little things, untidy things, annoy him. As another example, he wanted me to transfer money from his personal account to his iSaver account so that the amount in the iSaver account was "evened up". He likes round numbers so I transferred enough money from his personal account to his ISaver account to round up his iSaver account to an even number. He was very thankful.

He went to bed around 10 and Dianne went in to put in his eye drops. I was in the kitchen and heard her say goodnight to me but her voice was breaking. She closed the bedroom door and I heard her sobbing. I know that sound and understand only too painfully that feeling of the dreadful inevitable, that sense of all consuming loss; the fear, the loneliness. I didn't go down to see her, as I knew she wanted to be alone, as I do when those moments of absolute despair wash through me. We have discussed this and agreed that there is nothing we can do for each other in these moments of despair. We share that despair and are as one, but the pain of this is absolute and singularly individual and neither one of us can say that "it will be OK" because there is no OK anymore. We are two lost ships in the dark and together we are one lost ship in the dark. We can't help each other through this crisis other than through the knowledge that we are united in our love for each other and our children; we were together in the beginning and we will be together in the end.

A couple of minutes later I sent him a text 'goodnight' but he didn't respond. I waited another 5 minutes and then went in to see him but he was fast asleep.

Dianne had a restless night as she does most nights and that is a situation that we unavoidably and regretfully share.

Jack responded to my text of the night before:

6 March
3.36 am
Wellness 5/10

> **J** *all good*

Di said he was forgetful for most of the day but seemed to pick up in the afternoon. Uneventful in every other way.

He also had his Artesunate injection.

No change from yesterday but be is excited about Dianne's birthday tomorrow. I also reminded him that it will be 20 months since diagnosis so it was his special day too. He frowned and said, "Yeah, I know, but I still hate being like this". So do I Jack, so do I.

7 March
Wellness 6/10

Dianne had him out and about today as we want to get him moving and stimulated. However, he was very tired and slept a lot when he got home.

But the funny statistic is that even though today he complained of a small headache (Dianne gave him some Panadol at 5 pm), he has had no headaches over at least the last four days. This is unusual but good news and I will take any good news any day of the week.

He was in his room all night sitting on his bed. I went in to see him several times and he was content, watching a "TV show" on his computer and corresponding with friends on his mobile.

He is going to sleep now but complained of a small headache, so Di gave him a Panadol – he insisted on "one", not two tablets. It is ironic, with the toxic level of drugs he consumes daily that he would baulk at a couple of Panadol. I again reminded him that tomorrow was his 20th month since diagnosis and he laughed but said "I am sick of my shit problems". I said, "I know" and then blew him a kiss goodnight and went upstairs to finish my diary before I too go to bed.

8 March
Wellness 3/10

Another fragile beginning. He came upstairs around 8 am with Dianne's birthday present in his hand but looked like he had been crying. He said I have lost my memory again, so I would assume another complete wipe. He had remembered Dianne's birthday however as he checks his calendar every day when he wakes up. I said it is also special because today is 20 months post diagnosis for you but it paled into insignificance as he struggled with his brain. He smiled and said, "But I lost my memory again".

I rang Dianne late morning to see how he was and she said "fragile".

It was a lost day for Jack. He is very quiet and his voice weak. He laughs most times he speaks and that has become a new characteristic. His vulnerability is palpable and my heart breaks when I am alone and dwell on the shell of a boy that he is. I don't know if this is the quiet before the storm or the lowest point before we start to climb again. I know nothing but when alone I fear the worst. And I miss him as I sense his loneliness and despair and when I am in the office I want to be home, with him. Are we winning or losing and if we are losing, do we continue with all these medications or just fold up the tent and enjoy the chocolates and whisky as the days fade to grey and then black?

All night he has been showing Dianne and I the same pictures of jackets and caps that he likes and asks our opinion as he is considering buying them online. I have seen it 20 times since I have been at home. Dianne – many times more.

He is trapped in the endless cycle of despair and knowledge of who he once was ("I know I was very smart once") but frustrated by the fact that he can't remember the last 10 minutes, let alone the last 24 hours. Because of his memory issue and loss of processing skills, he is like a small child, not a man of 21. Jack has gone and I just want him back. My beautiful family of 8.

9 March

Wellness 4/10

Jack fragile and a little uncoordinated. No real change from yesterday, however we had a lively afternoon together with Di. I took Di to Frogmore Creek for lunch and Jack came too. We wouldn't ever leave him on his own.

I drove so Jack and Dianne enjoyed a glass of wine over lunch. He is aware of everything but continually apologises for "his bad brain".

Ash, Chris, Hugh and Jack played a couple of games in the evening.

10 March

Wellness 4/10

Ditto. However, he woke with a small nagging headache, which later went away with Panadol.

We took him to Hugh's football game and he went for a little walk with me around the park. He is fine and spends a lot of time chatting to friends on his phone and looking at stuff to buy – like luggage (?), shoes, jackets and caps.

He had a headache just before dinner but ate well. It was a warm night and we moved the dining table out onto the porch and fired up the barbecue. Unlike my father, I hate barbecuing as the cleaning drives me nuts and I always get the short straw.

Jack had salad and a pork chop and enjoyed the meal but appeared a little preoccupied.

After dinner he complained of a headache again so we suggested he rest on the couch. He fell asleep and woke about an hour later, feeling better. We decided he should have an early night and Dianne gave him a Melatonin tablet, which accelerated his tiredness even though with constant yawning he insisted that he wasn't tired!

He slept well.

11 March

Wellness 5/10

He woke with a small headache but was in good spirits.

I went down to see him in his room after breakfast and we chatted for a couple of minutes. He was very comfortable, sitting on his bed but didn't remember Hugh's game on Saturday.

He had a "weird" headache feeling around 6 when he came up for dinner. He also remembered Adrian's name (been referring to him as "my second oldest brother" for a couple of weeks) and recalled Adrian coming down here. He also remembered that the sweat top he had on ("Heartbreaker" across the front) was given to him by Adrian. He ate dinner and his head cleared.

We had a chat while I enjoyed a whisky and later he went to bed.

He came up to the kitchen around 7.30 am and said that he had a bit of a headache but it wasn't severe. It was on both sides of his temple but said it was really external, rather than internal. More so on his left side. He tried to explain that he wanted some toast but couldn't find the words. He also knew that he can't eat toast and joked about wanting it but knowing he can't have it. But we compromised and gave him half of a ketogenic bread roll (that I made previously) with bacon and eggs. He REALLY enjoyed that!!

His headache disappeared without taking any medication.

He had lunch – I made him salad with prawns and a rich creamy satay sauce. He really enjoyed it but then again, he says that about every meal. Never complains.

He went for a walk after I hounded him several times and then had a sleep.

Dianne cooked him lamb meatballs and salad for dinner. I hate lamb! So fatty, but Jack enjoyed it.

He has been in good humour all day and no recurrent headaches.

Playing Pop and Hop at the moment with Ash, Chris and Di. He has the biggest smile on his face and takes losing in his stride – with grace and humour.

Slight soreness in the back of the head when he woke up. Not unusual as has been a constant issue for several months. The pain is external and not a headache.

12 March
Wellness 7/10

13 March
Wellness 7/10

At least that was the way we interpreted it but it was internal and part of the dying process as the tumours were growing and crushing his brain.

He had a good day although his muddle-headedness has not improved. He constantly apologises for it and we retort that he has nothing to be sorry for and please do not ever apologise. NOT YOUR FAULT!

He had his Artesunate injection at Gore Street Medical.

I have been bashing my brain for ideas to give him something to do during the day as he is lost and bored, so I discussed learning the guitar. He said no, as his brain was mush and it was too hard. I bought a guitar anyway and he again said no. So I convinced Chris to have lessons (he was keen anyway) and teach Jack. Jack still reluctant but we will see how this plays out.

Had a whisky with me later in the evening and that made him tired so he went to bed.

14 March
Wellness 6/10

Repeat of yesterday. He is now stumbling with every second word and just can't find the word he is searching for. We have started to finish his sentences because he gets quite animated and clearly frustrated (although in a nice way) as he struggles to find words that are no longer there. He keeps repeating "my shit brain" and it is "the swelling, isn't it?".

I went down to talk to him tonight in his room after dinner and he was sitting quietly on the bed staring at the wall. I asked him what he was thinking and he said with a smile "I don't know; I can't remember; it is my shit brain; sorry". But he had the guitar in his room and said he really liked the look of it. It is a start.

Had some knee pain this morning but overall a good day. He only needed headache medication once and that was after he woke from an afternoon nap.

15 March
Wellness 7/10

I made him dinner at 6.20 pm, and after he had finished I convinced him to walk up and down the stairs a couple of times with 2x3 kg weights to get his body active. He does very little exercise although I remind him every day. He has lost so much muscle tone.

He spent the evening in his room but came upstairs around 9.30 and said he was really tired. Dianne gave him his Melatonin tablet and he went to bed.

Déjà vu.

16 March
Wellness 6/10

He was up early (I heard him when I got up to exercise at 5.30 am). He had pain, but not a headache and it was in the same spot at the back of the left side of his head. Said he had been lying there for several hours but didn't want to wake Dianne or me. I said he MUST wake us whenever he is uncomfortable (our bedroom door is never closed). I gave him two Panadol and two Nurofen and then gave him a Melatonin tablet. He went back to bed.

He had his Avastin injection. Uneventful in every other way but repeats probably 100 times a day: "I know it is frustrating as I don't remember too much".

I was still up at 2 am and he came upstairs and said he had some head pain. I gave him the usual 2 Panadol and 2 Nurofen and told him to take a Melatonin tablet, which he did, and then he went back to bed.

17 March
Wellness 6/10

Head pain (external) again, same spot, early morning. Di gave him the usual 2 Panadol and 2 Nurofen around 7 am. The

pain reappeared several times during the day and we repeated
(with at least a four-hour interval) the same 2+2.

After breakfast he went down to his room and looked
confused. Said his head was feeling funny "but in a good way".
I asked him to explain what he meant but he couldn't. I asked
him if he wanted to go and watch Chris and Hugh play football
against Olympia at 10 am and he said he would love to but just
needed to rest. I told Di to go on alone and if Jack improves

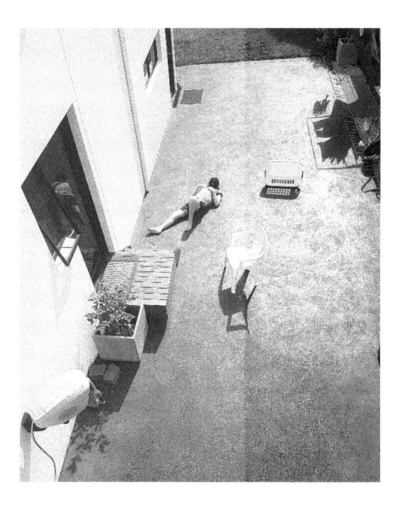

we will join her. He laid back on the bed and went to sleep. He woke about 30 minutes later and was fine but couldn't remember anything we had discussed.

"I know it is frustrating as I don't remember too much", started every conversation. But a really lost soul today. I got him to sit in the sun after he woke up from his nap and later he laid down on the concrete in the sun. After about 40 minutes I told him to come inside but he needed me to help him up. Quite feeble – could push him over with a feather. He shuffles around now like an old man. Breaks my heart if I dwell on it; it is numbing what that boy is going through.

But he smiles a lot so can be very pleasant company although memory issues no better and that situation could even have worsened.

Later two of his friends, Ed and Jackson, came over to spend time with him. They realised very quickly just how disorientated he was so the conversation became very simple and repetitive. Jack has such great friends. We had some whiskies, beer and wine and the boys ordered pizza – my shout!

They stayed to just after 8 pm and Jack went to bed around 10.

18 March
Wellness 5/10

Uneventful and same cycle. He remembered Ed and Jackson coming over when he woke up but later on forgot. He had several photos from the previous night of the three of them together and he would pull it out and say, "What's this? I don't remember."

Shuffling around the house all-day and lost. I try and talk to him as much as I can but he is confused about everything, even the fact that he has brain cancer. I reassure him and tell him he is doing well, that he is not alone and we love him. He appreciates that, but that memory evaporates as soon as I turn around.

He is tired a lot more and had another sleep after breakfast and again this afternoon. I was talking to him at 7.30 and he said he was tired. I told him that his body needs all the energy to fight the disease and he looked at me and said, "what disease?"

He went to bed at 10.15 pm, no head pain.

19 March
Wellness 5/10

I was up early and Jack came up to the lounge room and said his head was sore – same outside spot. I gave him a cup of coffee with cream – putting a lining on his stomach before I gave him some Nurofen. I then gave him 2 + 2. Dianne woke, and she took over. The head pain settled after a while and later he had breakfast.

I came home around 4 pm and he seemed fine. But if I was to be dispassionate (or let's call it "frank"), I think he is getting weaker and less stable on his feet. He holds the wall or the banister when he is going up and down the stairs. His forgetfulness is acute (in every meaning of the word). And today he slipped and fell heavily in the bathroom. I don't think he lost consciousness (i.e. blacked out) but he wears socks everywhere and the bathroom tiles are naturally slippery. However, in his weakened state he would easily lose his balance with any loss of friction. He hurt his knees but seemed OK after a few minutes.

We asked him if he wanted to play Pop and Hop but he declined. Seems less engaged and he does not usually make the effort to start a conversation but happy to respond if engaged.

But very difficult talking to him as nothing sinks in and a lot of what we say he struggles to comprehend.

He won't exercise although promises me every day that he will. He is so white, so pale, so frail and so wrecked. But I am not even sure that is a such a good idea as he struggles to get up the stairs and has little energy for even shuffling around the house. He is getting exhausted and his body has all the signs of being broken.

So when do you call it for what it is? The end?

I can kid myself sometimes that we are winning but winning what? I am not even sure what winning means anymore as a full, uncompromising recovery will never happen. Winning to me looks like he gets his memory back and starts to get fit again. Looks like he is on top of this rather than being crushed by it. Can I hope for anything else? Yes, but I don't think Jack has much time. He believes he is getting better, as that is an easy yarn to tell, as his spirits need inflating not deflating.

And if I have to sit with him in palliative care I just wish he was lucid so that we talk about everything in a mature way as we both face a terrible conclusion. But not like this, with him too compromised to really understand his fate and the thought of having to tell him the truth every 10 minutes is not a burden I want to contemplate, let alone carry. Yet it is a burden I will carry as he would carry for me.

He went to bed at 9.30 and commented even at 8.30 that he was tired. His usual spot head pain was back so he got 2+2 and also took his Melatonin tablet.

He is asleep now.

I was in Sydney for all of Tuesday but back today, Wednesday.

Di said that he woke yesterday morning with no head pain. However, so far today he has had the 2+2 three times.

She remarked that there has been a marked deterioration in his overall health over the last couple of days.

I now nod, no longer finding other (implausible) explanations to counter these observations.

He is sleeping a lot more and obviously tired a lot more. He asked me again tonight what was wrong with him.

I drove him to the Prince of Wales Hotel to catch his friends and I told him and his friends that he could have a couple of drinks – glass of whisky (he likes Makers Mark) and a glass of house pinot noir. But he told me at least twice, after we had the discussion, that he wouldn't drink as he didn't think it was good for him. So I told him again (and again), all good, have a couple of drinks and enjoy yourself! He was really looking forward to meeting his friends and they were tasked with looking after him (so the base was covered).

Di and I agreed that he might be too fragile to get an Uber home, so I went to the office (which is just around the corner from the pub) and that is where I am now, writing this and preparing for two Board meetings and one Finance Committee meeting over the next 48 hours.

So I am waiting for his call but have had several texts from him and he is really enjoying himself! So glad I talked him into going out.

Picking him up at 10.

When I got there, he was sitting unsteadily in a near empty bar with Jackson, his friend. They were talking to the barman. He had pain (usual spot) and was unsteady on his feet – think this time it was alcohol related.

Got him home and he had his usual 2+2 and then went to bed.

I spent the day in the office and rang Dianne mid-afternoon. She said he was generally good but very weak and had nearly collapsed at Harvey Norman (when she was with Jack in the electrical section) and again at the front door after she got him home.

22 March
Wellness 4/10

She also said that she had been reading a lot on Jack's (ailing) symptoms and was convinced he was close to the end. I didn't disagree with her and knew in my own mind that she was probably right. I got upset when I got off the phone – my newfound and unavoidable reality.

When I was driving home I wanted to see him and hug him and talk to him about the end. Let's at least have the discussion. So I sat with him and said what would you say if I told you that all that we are doing may not work and you may not have long to live? He said but it is working, isn't it and I just have a bit of swelling? I said you have been getting weaker over the last week and I am getting worried that maybe we are not winning anymore. He looked at me with the saddest look and said, "It is not good …?". I said maybe it is not good but we can't be sure. At this time Chris came upstairs and handed something to Jack. It was a plastic bag that had something in it. Here Dad, he said, "Happy birthday!"

It was a Liverpool Football Club top.

I cried.

We sat and had a glass of red wine together later and then he went to bed.

23 March

Wellness 4/10

I was up at 5.30 and texted Jack if he was OK. He sent me a thumb's up symbol (great way to start the day I thought).

I had an early morning Board meeting at Clifton Beach and left at 7.30 after I had been in to see him.

I was back at 11 am and at 12.30 we drove to the Royal for a meeting with Jack's oncologist.

Jack finds it difficult to answer questions and can look dazed and confused more often than not. It was obvious to John that his mental state had deteriorated. John gave him a number of tests for his reflexes, weighed him, reviewed his latest blood results, checked his blood pressure and his eyes, felt around his head and declared he was in perfect health! Shame about the tumour.

He later when upstairs for his Avastin injection and I picked up Di and Jack around 3.30 to take them home.

Due to our concerns, we decided to have another MRI and that is booked for Tuesday at 9.30 am. We need to be sure that we are not wasting our time with further treatments and maybe it is time for a reality check – stop treatments and plan move into palliative care. I am not expecting good news. No more bullshit Ken.

Due to his unsteadiness on his feet, I suggested we put a chair in the shower so that he could sit on it. He needs to be reminded to have a shower these days whereas before he would have at least one (and sometimes two) shower/s a day. I put a plastic chair in the shower just now and explained to him how to use it. I thought he might get upset but he just nodded and smiled. However, I told him that I didn't want to "cure your cancer to then have you bleed out on the bathroom floor because you have fallen through the shower screen". We have just renovated the bathroom and he has a big walk in shower with a frameless glass screen and it wouldn't be impossible to fall into it.

He just had a shower and came back upstairs with that same confused/dazed/lost look. Something is bothering him but he can't tell me what it is.

He was falling asleep around 9 pm on the couch (maybe helped by the dram of Japanese whisky I had given him earlier) so we put him to bed.

24 March
Wellness 2/10

I was in the lounge room at 1.30 am when he appeared in front of me. Said his knees were sore. I had some "cold" tape that I had bought recently for him, as this was a recurring problem. I wrapped both knees while he laid down on the couch and then I put a blanket on him as he was cold from the wrappings. After half an hour he said the pain had gone and so he went back to bed.

I came upstairs around 8 am and Jack was on the couch with Dianne. I asked him how he was and he said he was in pain. I looked at Dianne and she said, yes same spot and it just started and for which she had given him one codeine tablet. But he had woken up pain-free an hour earlier. He also had some minor (right) knee pain.

The pain eased to almost nothing by 9 am.

We were going to take him to Hugh's football game (Chris is injured) but he was very tired and he looked like he was going to have a sleep. I went to the game and came home around 2.30 pm and the first thing I saw as I walked up the stairs was Jack sitting on his bed, with the biggest smile on his face.

He is sleeping now.

He had some problems with his right eye and almost lost vision in that eye for part of the day.

He came upstairs later and seemed alright, however early evening he looked more dazed than usual. We decided to keep a close eye on him. He was resting and watching his computer and looking at his phone on the couch in the sunroom. Dianne and I were next door in the lounge room. I saw him get up and he staggered as he went for the stairs. I jumped up and ran around the corner but he was half way down the stairs and he dropped his computer. By this time Dianne had grabbed him from behind and I picked up the computer and we walked him gingerly down the stairs where he promptly laid down on his bed. He closed his eyes and said he felt funny. I told Di to leave him and I will sit with him. He saw me sitting there and would open his eyes, gave me a weak smile and then close his eyes again. He looked very weak and exhausted. After about 10 minutes he opened his eyes, smiled and said I am OK now Dad, all good. I said just close your eyes and rest and I will let you have a little sleep. He said, "Sure, thanks, I am OK" (again).

Di and I didn't speak but we looked at each other. There was nothing to say and we both knew what was on each other's mind – running out of time.

We later had a discussion about how this will end and we both conceded that there was definite movement in the brain – the eyes, the odd (new feelings), the unsteadiness, the staggered walking stride, the increased frequency of head pain. We just hope that it will be quick and not drawn out as he is suffering.

He later came upstairs and he was a lot better and even asked for a whisky, which I gladly indulged him.

He went to bed around 10.

I heard him moving around at 4.30 am so I got up to see what he was doing. He was dressed and upstairs. I said what are you doing, and he said he couldn't sleep. I said no pain? And he said no, all good, just couldn't sleep.

I left him on the couch and went back to bed, however checked on him about an hour later and he was sound asleep.

He didn't have a headache all day until around 6 pm, after we woke him from a very long nap. We went to Yum Cha at 11 am and were home at 12.30. Jack went to sleep almost straight away.

25 March
Wellness 4/10

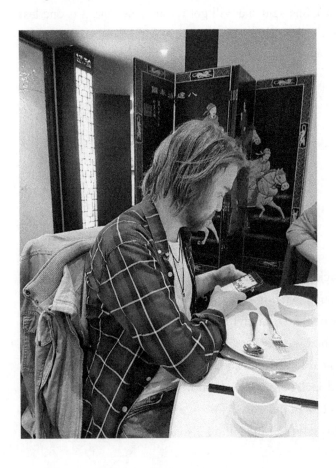

Di said quietly to me at Yum Cha that Jack wanted to pay for lunch. I said it will be expensive but Di said he was very insistent so even if he forgets you should remind him. When the bill came, he pulled out his credit card and gave it to me with the biggest smile on his face. "It is mine," he said.

I have just made his ketogenic rolls and waiting for them to cook in the oven. Jack is up and Di has just walked him downstairs. She is laughing with him. His headache has gone.

She also just told me that there is a wheelchair being provided to us from the Whittle Ward (Palliative Care Ward at the Royal). She said she will get it tomorrow and it is one less worry due to his weakening and unsteady nature.

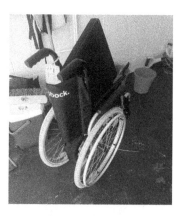

Jack was very sleepy after dinner and later went to sleep on the couch. After he awoke, he sat next to Di and went to sleep again. We woke him at 10 pm and Di walked him downstairs and into bed.

The rolls are cool and I have put them away but not before I showed Jack before he went down to bed. Look great he said and then closed his eyes.

It is now 11.15 pm and I also am going to bed.

I heard him get up around 2.30 am and went to see if he as all right. He was just up to go to the toilet but said he was fine and went back to bed. When I finished exercising at 8.20 am he was in the lounge room with Di. She said he was fine, no head pain but slight knee pain.

I came home around 4.30 pm and Di said she had given him his first 2+2 but nothing else all day.

Palliative Care rang around 5 pm to ask how he is and Di spoke to the doctor. They sense it is close as we relayed what we are now experiencing. These are classic symptoms.

I went in to see him and later he fell asleep on the bed. He came up for dinner at 6.20 pm (pumpkin soup with cream) and appeared OK but shortly thereafter he complained of head pain and Di gave him the usual 2+2. After dinner he sat with us in the lounge room and was on his mobile phone for a short time before he fell into a deep sleep. Di roused him to see if he was OK and he just mumbled that he was very tired and promptly went back to sleep. It is 9 pm and he is still asleep in the lounge room.

We woke him and Di walked him down the stairs at 9.30 pm. He is exhausted.

Tomorrow at 9.30 am he has his MRI and I think it will be his last. I have written him off so many times before and then we find a get-out-of-gaol-free card. But he has never been so energy depleted and mentally exhausted as he is now. Life is going through some repetitive motions and he believes all the pain and suffering is worth it because he is getting better. I wish it was. I wish!

And if the MRI is benign, how do we explain this shit?!!

It is 10.10 pm and I am exhausted as I didn't sleep at all last night as my mind wouldn't let go of what life will be like when he is gone. Couldn't let go. That testimonial, the faces, the tears and the coffin. Over and over and over and over it played.

27 March

Wellness 4/10

I didn't come home till late on Tuesday night and Jack was asleep. Jack had his MRI earlier in the day and seemed OK but unsteady on his feet and feeble. The radiologist held his arm and walked him into the change room. He appreciated the support although looked a little embarrassed and gave a weak smile.

This is the future.

On Wednesday I reviewed his medications sheet (we write everything down–which meds and time) and there were three periods when he had medications for head pain/headaches.

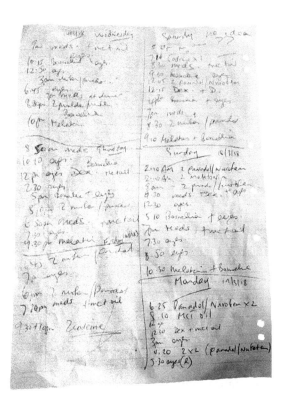

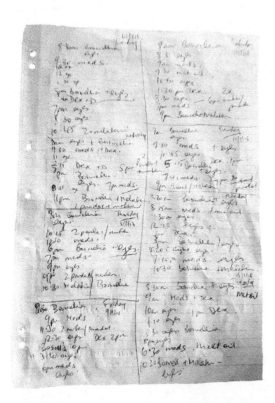

It is now 11.21 am and I am sitting with him while he sleeps on the couch. He hasn't said much this morning other than to tell us that he has severe head pain. We have given him some pills and he has been asleep for about an hour in the lounge room.

We got a call from Victoria, asking us to come in today at 3 pm to discuss Jack's MRI results. We knew what to expect and Dianne said it is not easy (or fair) dragging Jack around so we would prefer a phone call. John rang at 12.45 and confirmed that all the news was bad and there was extensive progression of the tumour/s and there was nothing

28 March

Wellness 3/10

we could do to stop it from ending his life in 3-6 weeks. He recommended immediate cessation of the Avastin infusions as they were doing little or no good and it was only (possibly) prolonging the inevitable. Below is a copy of my hand-written note I made during the call.

I tried to talk to him about the phone call after I got home at 5 but he smiled at me and closed his eyes and was clearly very drowsy. I just sat next to him and watched him fall in and out of sleep over the next 30 minutes.

I managed to get him into the shower before dinner (he still showers on his own).

We decided to end the ketogenic dietary restrictions as they make no sense now and he might as well enjoy some of his favourite foods in the little time he has left. So, he had his first piece of garlic bread in nearly two months. Now that went down well!

He was very tired at 8.15 pm after Di gave him an Endone and we walked him downstairs and Dianne tucked him into bed. He is asleep now.

I have told his four closest friends (we have set up a WhatsApp group site) and they are all shattered. They have told his other friends.

Two of the boys – Ed and Nick – had previously arranged to come over tomorrow night and Jack was looking forward to it. So am I.

Usual day for Jack, sleeping a lot and a string of headaches. Occupational therapy staff visited us and we have a couple of walkers and a toilet assistance contraption. On the latter, Jack

29 March
Wellness 2/10

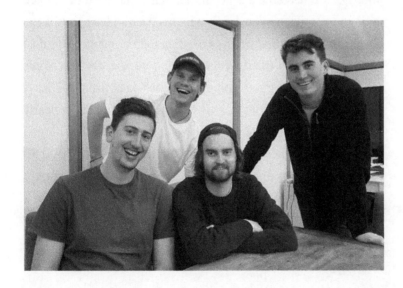

very unhappy with it and insisted that we remove it which we have since done.

Ed, Nick Burk and Jackson came out to see Jack at 5.30. Jackson joined at the last minute. He was visibly very happy to see them but became teary-eyed when he found he couldn't express his thoughts. The boys clearly very sympathetic and a bit teared up later in the evening. They left around 8 and Jack went to bed soon after, very tired. We also now have just filled a prescription for methadone and he took his first (quarter tablet).

He woke up around 3 am and went to the toilet. I jumped up to see if he was OK and when he saw me he said "bloody hell" with a big smile on his face. I said are you OK and he said fine, no problems.

30 March
Wellness 2/10

He woke around 9 with a bad headache and Dianne gave him some codeine. He went back to sleep and he roused around midday. Still had a headache and felt nauseous. Said he wanted to go to the toilet and he sat up with his head in his hands, head bowed and eyes closed. He was like that for 5 minutes then rolled back on the bed. I finally got him to sit up and got him to the toilet. Dianne said I was going to stay but Jack insisted I leave as he said he was OK to do this. He was in the toilet for nearly half an hour and then he asked me to come in. He was sitting in a seat in front of the washbasin and said to me. "I am confused". I washed his hands and then he went upstairs. He wasn't hungry but he needed food with his medications so Dianne gave him a sliver of pizza and some salad. He ate it reluctantly.

He then went into the lounge room and laid down. Dianne gave him a small piece of chocolate and as I was making the chocolate Easter eggs (as I do every Easter) I took a jelly snake into him. He looked at it and then at me and said, "I can't eat this can I?"

I said yes you can. He looked worried and said "I can't as it not on my diet". So I said, "Jack your diet is not working so yes you can". He looked very worried and stared at me and said, "Not working?". At that point Dianne saw the worry on his face and heard the fear in his voice and said, "Well Jack you can have a little, because it is Easter, but only a little". He seemed to accept that and ate the snake with the most satisfied look on his face.

We can't tell him. His head is screwed as it is and that would only add to his perplexity and fear.

We know all this sugar is feeding the cancer but we have starved it and it still is growing so he might as well die happy. And we both hope he goes quickly as he has no quality of life and if we can't beat it then we want to save him from any further suffering. It destroys us watching him like this, as this foreign thing strips him of his humanity and dignity.

I managed to get him into the shower and when he finished he asked me to dry his hair. I dried it and combed it and remembered doing that when he was a little boy.

He came back upstairs and sat back on the couch. When Dianne offered him a bit of the rocky road chocolate I had made he baulked and said, "I can't eat that?".

He has lost his appetite but we gave him a small bowl of bolognaise with some pasta which he enjoyed.

We walked him to bed around 9 pm.

31 March
Wellness 1/10

Very emotional morning. Dianne and I beside ourselves and in a world of hurt. Tears stained every part of the morning and extended across the day.

He woke with severe pain (which is the norm now) and Di gave him two Endone tablets. She managed to also get him to the toilet and he went back to bed and fell asleep.

I went in and sat with him around 10. He sensed I was in the room and opened his eyes. I smiled and he smiled back and then closed his eyes again.

It is now 11.15 and he is still in pain.

I have just rung Turnbull Funerals to discuss Jack's funeral and cremation. Not an easy phone call but I know nothing about the process, options, timing, organisation and everything else that goes with the end of life. And I know emotionally, it is beyond Dianne. I have a meeting with Peter O'Brien on Tuesday at 10.30 am.

Dianne got Jack up around 3 pm and sat him in a chair next to the window in the lounge room. It was a very warm day and the heat from the window made me feel uncomfortable but with the medications Jack is on he is usually cold, regardless of the temperature.

He was in and out of consciousness for most of the evening while he laid down on the lounge next to where I was sitting. Dianne sat next to me. Every so often he would open his eyes and turn his head to see if we were there and then reach for his phone, ask us to read his messages and then agree a response, which Dianne typed in for him. He would play on his phone for several minutes and then it would slip from his hand as he went back to sleep.

We got him to bed around 10 pm but not before we got him to the toilet. Dianne held him from behind with her eyes closed and I turned my back and he faced the toilet and urinated. There are other times when he insists on being left alone during these times and he waves his hand and says "go away". But not tonight and I think it was because he was exhausted.

He then sat dutifully in the chair and Dianne washed his hands and brushed his teeth.

We then tucked him into bed and both kissed him, knowing there is every possibility that one day soon he might not wake up and every 'goodnight' could be in reality 'goodbye'.

APRIL

1 April

Wellness 2/10

We heard him go to the bathroom around 6.30 am and Dianne jumped up out of bed. When I came upstairs around 7.30 he was sitting on the couch in the lounge room and Di said he was good this morning. I said "good morning" and he said "I am in a lot of pain". Threw Di as he hadn't mentioned it before. So she gave him one codeine.

It is now 8.45 and Dianne has escorted him downstairs to have a nap in his room, which he wanted.

I left a little after 10 to fill a prescription for codeine for Jack. Our usual chemist was closed so I went to Rosny (about 12 minutes away). In Hobart, 12 minutes is an effort but in Sydney it would take you that long to get out of your driveway!

We were low on codeine so we had to get some today.

I gave the prescription to the chemist and she read it and walked away. After two minutes she came back and said that there was a problem and I had to get the prescription filled at the Amcal at Shoreline (where I had just been). I said it was closed and she said she couldn't help me as they (Amcal) had stuffed up the prescription by linking several prescriptions with the codeine. I didn't understand what she was talking about and she said that the Federal Government is very strict on codeine now and putting that with other prescriptions was a problem.

The codeine prescription had been stapled to a prescription for Keppra but I was none the clearer or wiser.

She was very pleasant and clearly and equally exasperated. I said it was for my son, Jack, who had brain cancer and was at home in pain. I suggested she ring the Royal and talk to the oncologist on duty to clarify, which she promptly did. I sat down and suddenly the enormity of what I was getting and why I was here and the fact that I had tell a stranger about the terminal health of my son overwhelmed me. I tried to stop it but I broke down.

The pharmacist and the attendant – two middle-aged women – understood all too well my emotional outburst and were very kind and sympathetic. For my part I felt embarrassed but what can you do? I didn't choose to have a son with terminal brain cancer and sure as would prefer to be in the garden than here almost begging for a script to be filled because my son was in pain. And you stop and feel you are taking control and then bang, off you go again.

I apologised and of course they wouldn't hear of it and even opened a new box of tissues for me. The box on the counter was half full but I think they were thinking there were some serious floodgates about to be tested and breached!

I got the script and came home.

Jack was sitting next to Di with a patch over his right eye – it sometimes helps when he has problems with that eye but he looked relaxed and calm.

Di said he was a lot more lucid and with it than yesterday.

A better day in a sea of bad days …

It is now 3 pm and he has just woken from a long nap. He is on his phone and gave me a smile. Million-dollar smiles.

I did some weeding this afternoon and my next-door neighbour, Matt said 'hello'. He, as well as our other neighbours, know about Jack. He asked me how we were travelling and I said not great. He said if there is anything we can do, let me know. When he first found out he brought around a huge lasagne, which the boys and Dianne still talk about. He was a chef. I said well there was that lasagne ... He said consider it done! Just then one of his boys, Sam (who I think is 6 or 7?) said hello and asked me if I got any chocolate for Easter. I said I don't eat chocolate anymore but as a matter of fact I made some for Easter for the boys and asked him if he would like some? He said "yes". I said do you have any allergies and he said in a very loud voice with a big smile on his face "I don't have any allergies!!". I said OK, I will bring around some special chocolate this afternoon (that I made over Easter) for you and Ben (his younger brother).

I got my Matthew to take a chocolate bunny around to Sam and Ben after I came inside.

About an hour later we heard the doorbell and Matt was there with several ice cream containers of food – Thai pumpkin soup and chilli beef and bean pasta bake. Di answered the door and she was overwhelmed. She thanked Matt with tears streaming down her face.

He had a small dinner and a small glass of pinot noir which he drank over 90 minutes. At around 7.30 he said he was tired and Dianne said it is too early to go to sleep now, so how about you have a nap on the couch?

He was restless and at 7.45 pm it was obvious that he needed to go to bed. Usual drill – Di in bathroom and after teeth brushed and in bed shorts I kissed him goodnight.

I was up in the kitchen looking at some old home videos at 9.45 pm when I heard him stir. I have been trying to pull together a collage of Jack's life, as I will use it to reflect on his wonderful (but short) life at his funeral. And I have to think about this, as it is the unavoidable reality of our fate. Locked in, cancer wins, next!!

I went downstairs and he was in the bathroom and I heard him urinating. When he came out of the toilet he was dressed and I asked him what he was doing as he should be in bed. He said "no" and showed me his phone (speaking is becoming more difficult and he is increasingly incoherent). When I opened his phone a reminder came up about the Arsenal Stoke game and now it all made sense.

However it is not on TV but Chris has an Optus login and he can run the game from his PC to the computer. But one problem, Chris is not at home as he is at the gym. So I am sitting here in the kitchen while Jacks sleeps on the couch and Chris is somewhere between here and Zap! Shit, shit, shit!!

Chris home at 10.15 and told Jack he will have a shower and then put the game on (which he said starts in 15 minutes).

While I am sitting here (10.25) I heard Jack say, "Now I understand". I went in to see him and asked him what he understands and he showed me his phone: Arsenal vs Stoke.

Now 10.31 and Chris in the lounge room and putting the game on.

10.40 I went in to see Jack as he was trying to talk to Chris but was incoherent. Jack looked at me and rubbed his head. I touched his head and said "pain?" He said "yes".

I spoke to Dianne who had gone to bed earlier and she said give him two Panadol and two Nurofen (which I did). He later complained that he couldn't see (eyes are failing) so I pulled a chair up close to the TV (which Chris was using to stream the game through) and helped him walk to it. He said that it was "better".

At half time he tried to get out of the chair but couldn't get the leverage. I helped him and walked him down the stairs and into bed.

Woke up around 8 with a very bad headache. Dianne got him upstairs and gave him two codeine tablets. He went to sleep on the couch.

2 April

Wellness 1/10

He is weaker and less stable on his feet.

I spent the day working through the old videos and identifying timelines to create a montage on that fateful day when we all say our final farewell. I want his funeral to be a celebration of his life, not dwell on his untimely death. We have that pain to bear separately for an eternity.

Afternoon was in and out of sleep on the couch. He is eating sparingly and still stuck on his diet –"Can I eat that?", "I can't eat that can I?".

We were planning catching up with Jack's friends at Shippies tonight at 5 but early afternoon it was obvious to me that he wasn't up for it. I told them and they were disappointed and asked, if not possible for Jack to go out (and I think that door is closed), could they come over in small group over the next couple of days?

I said maybe but he stresses as he can't talk and he feels embarrassed and I am not sure it is good for him right now. Tears were streaming down his face on Thursday night when Nick, Jackson and Ed came over to see him and he couldn't get the words out. He doesn't need the stress, yet his friends have every right to see him no matter how bad he is and have the chance to say goodbye. It is a dichotomy I will ponder over the next couple of days.

And then he got a message from Olivia – a girl that he was close to and who he pushed away when he was diagnosed. She obviously had heard from her peers about Jack's precarious health and was desperate to come out and see him. We asked him and he made it very clear that he didn't want her to see him like this. We asked him several times and he mumbled "not like this". Understood my son, understood.

We asked him if other friends could come out to see him and he repeated the same (unmistakable) syllable: "No".

He is in the lounge room at the moment with Di (it is 8.10 pm) and on his phone. Never sure what he does but it looks like he plays a couple of games, one being pool.

We will get him to bed soon.

We are talking to the district nurse tomorrow about home visits and palliative care on Thursday to have him assessed for when he takes that final step, never to return home. It will be a relief in one sense because as his pain builds, we can't keep him comfortable. However, he won't understand where he is and why he is there and that will break my heart every time we have that (endless) conversation. He is also always looking for his brothers (again asking today where they were). But what do you do? How many parents are facing the same heart-wrenching dilemma right now in this country? Hundreds … thousands?

He is getting tired so will probably get him to bed soon.

3 April
Wellness 1/10

I woke up early to exercise (5.30 am). On my phone was another message from Olivia.

< **Olivia** ☏ ⋮

Mon, 2 Apr. 2018 11:57 pm

Ken, thank you so much for your message. Sorry
for taking this long to get back to you, it's taken me
a while to process. I love your son so much, and he
knows that, but it would mean a lot to me for you to
remind him how much I love him. If you can pass
on a message from me, please just tell him a proper
goodbye from me, tell him that he's still going to be
my valentine next year, that I think he is the strongest
person I know, and that I'm so grateful to have had
this much extra time with him. I love him so much.
I'm more than happy to be in charge of organising
a wake for him at shippies when it comes time to
put that together, he's told me before that that's
what he's wanted, so I think he'd be comforted to
know that we'll do it and that it'll be a great day
of celebrating his life.
My heart is breaking for you and your family, I want
you to know that I'm thinking of you and willing
to do anything else to help ease pain that you,
Dianne, and your family must be feeling. You raised
someone very special and should be very proud
of yourselves. Olivia x

It was a beautiful message and opened the floodgates, which set the mood for the rest of the day. I showed Dianne and it set off a chain reaction.

It was in response to a message that she had sent Jack begging to come over and see him but he refused. I explained that to Olivia and added that he is just embarrassed. Her response was poignant and beautiful.

I was upstairs doing some stretches when I heard Jack's bathroom door close. I then heard 'bang' and rushed downstairs. I tried to get in the bathroom but Jack was slumped on the floor against the door. When I finally got him and lifted him up he seemed alright, but a little dazed.

I went to meet the funeral director and discuss Jack's funeral. I held it together pretty well but not a good moment when Dianne and I sat down later at home to discuss his casket – style, design and cost. I am not sure how many more emotional strands I have left.

And tonight, déjà vu, same bathroom, same place, same fall, same dazed boy.

We got him upstairs around 6 and back on the couch on the lounge room. Dianne put a small plate of food together for him and he said, "What is the point?"

I later read him Olivia's message but when I asked him if he knew who she was he said, "I don't remember". So I read part of the message. He looked bemused and then smiled. "Could you thank her for me?"

The palliative care doctor came out today and said he probably had a week (?) before he would have to move to palliative care. She increased his methadone dosage and he is now either unconscious (for most of the day) or *non compos mentis* when he is awake. He is asleep now in his bedroom.

Di just came up and said she just wished he would die in his sleep. And sadly, I agree. What is the point?

4 April
Wellness 2/10

I was dozing very early morning and heard Dianne scream and leap out of bed "Ken! Jack is moving". I jumped out of bed and at our bedroom door was Jack, leaning up against the wall. As Di and I came across him he looked shocked and didn't seem to know where he was going. He started to walk to our bathroom and Di said did you want to go to the toilet and he said "no, been". He then said "both" but neither of us were sure what he meant by it. We got him back into bed and he slept.

I went back to the funeral home today and confirmed the coffin we wanted and flower arrangement.

He had a reasonably good day – communicative a little more and we managed to shower him.

He ate well (like a sparrow but better than not eating at all).

Been asleep now for an hour (it is 7.45 pm).

5-7 April
Wellness 1/10

Each day the same – Jack getting weaker, disorientated, tired and sleeps a lot. Typical day we would help him go to the toilet in the morning, as he couldn't walk on his own, plus he fell over in the bathroom on two occasions.

Dianne is also now getting up at around 3 am and moving into Jack's room to help him go to the toilet if he wakes up early and we do not hear him.

On Saturday 7 April he vomited several times and we knew it wouldn't be long as this was one of the final signs of his body closing down.

8 April
Wellness 0/10

He threw up in the morning and couldn't keep anything down, notable including his pills. Dianne called an ambulance and went with them to Calvary. I saw them leave and said goodbye to Jack as it drove passed the house as I knew he wouldn't be coming home again. At least not alive.

Dianne rang several hours later and said he was stable and was being admitted to the Gibson Unit of St John's Hospital. It is the palliative care unit and his final resting place. Now it was just time.

13 April

Wellness 0/10

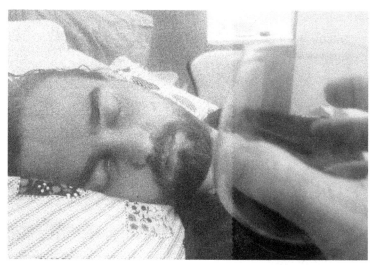

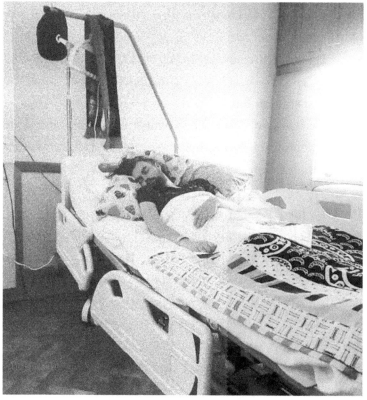

Today, ironically, is 22 months post diagnosis. A new record Jack!

I stayed with him in the evenings, sleeping uncomfortably on a bunk bed and Dianne took the day shift, so that one of us was with him always. I would go home after Dianne came in and sleep and continue working on my video and photo montages in preparation for Jack's funeral.

FINAL DAYS

Jack died at 1.45 pm on 15 April, a cold, wet Sunday afternoon. His breathing was rapid and had been for several days but in the last 10 minutes it eased and was normal, peaceful.

I was still hoping for a miracle and thought just maybe you had reached the bottom and were now coming back up.

It wasn't to be.

You had tears in your eyes and that will haunt me for the rest of my life because in that moment I think you knew this was the end and you were sad for all of us, and maybe for yourself.

Adrian, Matthew, Chris, Hugh, Mum and I were there. Stefan had said goodbye a couple of days earlier and was on his way back from Perth. However, you couldn't wait. You just stopped breathing. My beautiful son. One minute you were there and the next you were not.

When everybody left I stayed behind to say my final goodbye and I spoke to you for 10 minutes. I just wanted to say again, as I had said many times before, thank you for being my son and allowing me to enjoy the short but wonderful years of your precious life.

funeral

THE FUNERAL WAS HELD ON FRIDAY 20 APRIL AT 10 am at Turnbull Funerals in North Hobart. We reckon there were over 100 people there, including about 60 of your school friends and mates. I spoke, as did Chris, Kate Baldry and Joe Cairns (from Friends) and Jackson. I had also put together a photomontage and about 30 minutes of old (and recent) videos, which I thought reflected well on the adventures and misadventures of your wonderful (but oh so short) life. There was not a dry eye in the house but a few laughs during the videos. So many people were affected by your death and continue to be to this day and well beyond.

For Mum and me, the pain is as bad today as it was when you left us. Time has not healed this wound.

This is how we laid out the morning and I think you would have been chuffed Jack, particularly listening to Chris and Jackson recount their many memories of you.

And these were the handwritten notes on what songs you would have liked played at your funeral. I think you would have enjoyed the music:

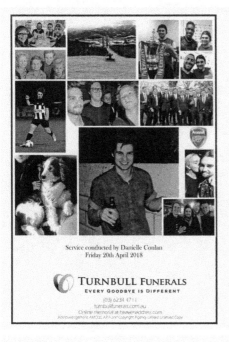

Service conducted by Danielle Conlan
Friday 20th April 2018

TURNBULL FUNERALS
EVERY GOODBYE IS DIFFERENT

(03) 6234 4711
turnbullfunerals.com.au
Online memorial at heavenaddress.com
Acknowledgements AMCOS, APRA and Copyright Agency Limited Licensed Copy

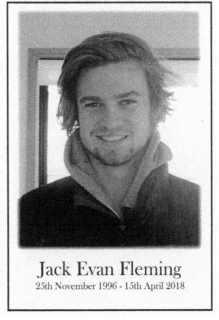

Jack Evan Fleming
25th November 1996 - 15th April 2018

Do Not Stand at My Grave and Weep

Do not stand at my grave and weep,
I am not there. I do not sleep.
I am a thousand winds that blow.
I am the diamond glints on snow.
I am the sunlight on ripened grain.
I am the gentle autumn rain.
When you awaken in the morning's hush
I am the swift uplifting rush
Of quiet birds in circled flight.
I am the soft stars that shine at night.
Do not stand at my grave and cry;
I am not there. I did not die.

Mary Elizabeth Frye

Order of Service

Opening Music
"Hey There Delilah" by Plain White T's

Welcome and Introduction
Danielle Conlan

Reflections of Jack's Life
Ken Fleming

Jack's Family Album
"One More Light" by Linkin Park
"Lost In The Supermarket" by The Clash
"Hey There Delilah" by Plain White T's
"I Won't Give Up" by Jason Mraz
"With Me" by Sum 41
"Hey Jude" by The Beatles
"In My Life" by The Beatles

Tribute to Our Brother
Chris Fleming

Video Compilation

Tributes to Jack
Kate Baldry Joe Cairns, The Friends' School
Jackson Nugent

Closing Words and Committal

Closing Music
"I Won't Give Up" by Jason Mraz
"One More Light" by Linkin Park

One More Light - Linkin Park
All Lost in ~~the~~ Clash supermarket
Hey There Delilah - Plain White T's
I wont give up - Jason Mraz
with Me
Hey Jude - Sum 41
The Life.

The Clash

My testimonial was this:

JACK'S FINAL DAY

THIS IS ONE OF THE HARDEST DAYS OF MY LIFE.

I WOULD PREFER TO BE ANYWHERE ELSE BUT SO WOULD JACK, SO HERE WE ARE.

SUNDAY 15 APRIL 2018 WAS THE WORST DAY.

DIANNE AND I WERE MARRIED IN MARCH 1996 AND JACK WAS BORN 9 MONTHS LATER, ON 25 NOVEMBER 1996.

THAT WAS NO COINCIDENCE AS WE HAD BEEN TRYING FOR THREE YEARS TO HAVE A BABY AND FINALLY JACK DECIDED TO JOIN US.

HE DIED, 21 YEARS LATER AFTER A 22 MONTH STRUGGLE WITH BRAIN CANCER.

HE WAS DIAGNOSED ON 8 JULY 2016 WITH GLIOBLASTOMA MULTIFORME BRAIN CANCER (GBM) WHICH IS ALWAYS GRADE 4 (I.E. TERMINAL/NO CHANCE/ FINISHED/YOU ARE OUT OF HERE).

HE WAS GIVEN 12 MONTHS TO LIVE BUT SURVIVED 22 MONTHS AFTER TWO MAJOR BRAIN SURGERIES, RADIATION THERAPY, ENDLESS ROUNDS OF DRUGS AND TREATMENTS, INCLUDING CHEMOTHERAPY.

IF HE HAD HEAD PAIN, HE WOULD SWALLOW – WITH ALL HIS MEDICATIONS – UP TO 20 PILLS A DAY.

EVERY DAY.

WE HAVE MORE DRUGS IN OUR HOME THAN MOST CHEMISTS!

WE MADE THE '60S LOOK TAME.

BUT HE NEVER CRIED, GAVE UP, OR SAID NO MORE.

I DID MY SHARE OF CRYING FOR HIM, AS DID HIS MUM. AS DID ALL OF US.

I ASKED HIM COUNTLESS TIMES AFTER EVERY BAD MRI, DO YOU WANT TO GIVE UP AND PARTY? ENJOY THE TIME YOU HAVE LEFT?

AND HE ALWAYS SAID, "NO DAD, NEVER."

"I HAVE TO SURVIVE TO HELP MY YOUNGER BROTHERS GROW UP AND GUIDE THEM."

WE HAD MANY INTIMATE AND CONFRONTING CONVER- SATIONS.

AND HE KNEW HE WAS PROBABLY NOT GOING TO MAKE IT.

HE ACCEPTED IT. DIANNE AND I REFUSED.

AND THE LETTERS HE WROTE IN DECEMBER AND WE HAVE JUST NOW RECEIVED AND READ, PROVE IT.

AND WE STILL DO.

THE FIRST CONFRONTING MOMENT WAS ON SATURDAY, 9 JULY 2016 (THE DAY AFTER HIS DIAGNOSIS), WHEN HE CAME UP FROM HIS ROOM EARLY EVENING AND SAID, "WHAT DOES THIS MEAN?"

"I WILL NEVER FINISH UNIVERSITY, HAVE A CAREER OVERSEAS, GET MARRIED, HAVE CHILDREN?"

AND WE SAID, "THAT IS EXACTLY WHAT THIS MEANS."

BUT THERE WERE TIMES WE THOUGHT WE HAD A CHANCE AND WHILE THERE WAS THAT SMALL SLIVER OF HOPE, HE SAID, "I WANT TO LIVE, NO MATTER WHAT I HAVE TO DO."

SO, WE FOUGHT ON AND LOOKED FOR ANOTHER DOOR TO OPEN.

AND LOOK WE DID – UNDER EVERY ROCK, DOWN EVERY RABBIT HOLE, ALONG EVERY CRAWL SPACE TRYING TO SOLVE THE UNSOLVABLE.

HE WAS ONE OF SIX SONS – DIANNE'S FIRST AND MY THIRD.

AND HE JUST HAD HIS SHIT TOGETHER FROM DAY ONE. JUST GOT ON WITH LIFE WITH LITTLE FUSS, NOISE OR MESS.

HIS PARENTS WERE JUST ALONG FOR THE RIDE, BUT HE WAS DOING THE DRIVING.

YOU WOULD SIT HIM IN THE CORNER WITH A PUZZLE, AND HE WOULD SIT FOR HOURS CONTENTED IN HIS OWN COMPANY.

AND HE WOULD NEVER CRY. AS HE DIDN'T HAVE TIME TO CRY AS THERE WAS SO MUCH INTERESTING STUFF TO DO AND DISCOVER.

BUT I FAILED HIM.

I PROMISED HIM I WOULD:
- GET HIM BACK DRIVING AGAIN – I DIDN'T;
- GET HIM BACK TO UNIVERSITY TO FINISH HIS DEGREES – I DIDN'T;
- GET HIM TO FALLS AT THE END OF THIS YEAR – I DIDN'T; AND
- SAVE HIS LIFE – I COULDN'T.

BUT I DID SAY TO HIM IF ANYONE CAN FIGURE OUT A WAY TO WALK OUT OF THE PALLIATIVE CARE UNIT WITH ME, IT WOULD BE HIM.

BUT IT DIDN'T HAPPEN.

HE HAD SEVERAL WORDS HE WANTED TO SAY TO HIS BROTHERS:

FIRSTLY, HE WAS GLAD IT WAS HIM AND NOT ONE OF THEM AS HE FELT HE WAS THE STRONGEST.

SECONDLY, HE SAID THAT THIS MUST NOT STOP ANY OF THEM FROM ACHIEVING ALL THEIR GOALS AND

HE WANTED THEM TO GO ON AND DO ALL THE THINGS HE COULDN'T DO.

AND NOW WON'T DO.

SO, HEED THOSE SENTIMENTS BOYS. AND THAT GOES FOR HIS MATES.

MAKE LIFE COUNT.

AND EVERY TIME YOU ACHIEVE SOME MILE-STONE, THINK OF JACK.

I HAVE A LOT OF PEOPLE TO THANK, INCLUDING STAFF AT CALVARY, THE ROYAL, ST JOHN'S, HIS NEUROSURGEON, HIS CLOSE AND LOYAL FRIENDS, THE TASMANIAN AMBULANCE SERVICE AND MY FAMILY AND FRIENDS.

HOWEVER, I WILL LEAVE THOSE PERSONAL NOTES FOR ANOTHER TIME.

BUT I DO NOT WANT TO DWELL ANYMORE ON JACK'S UNTIMELY DEATH BUT FOCUS OH HIS SHORT BUT WONDERFUL LIFE.

I WANT TO START WITH A MONTAGE OF PHOTOS THAT ARE INTENTIONALLY OUT OF SEQUENCE AS THAT IS THE WAY WE REMEMBER JACK.

AND LATER SOME VIDEOS THAT SHOW SOME OF HIS DYNAMIC AND INFECTIOUS CHARACTER.

FINALLY, ON A HAPPIER NOTE, THERE WILL BE A WAKE AT SHIPPIES IN BATTERY POINT ON SATURDAY, 28 APRIL, STARTING AT 6 PM. IT IS WHAT JACK WANTED AND MY ONLY DISAPPOINTMENT IS THAT JACK WON'T BE THERE.

THANK YOU.

the end

I NEVER WANTED TO WRITE THIS BUT HERE I AM,
Sunday 29 April 2018. You are dead. Stopped breathing at
1.45 pm on 15 April 2018, just over 22 months since diagnosis. I
am sitting in your room, at your desk, writing this final chapter
of your short life, my son. You were given 12 months and we
got 22 but it didn't change the outcome, did it?

I have never known pain like this – it is unrelenting and
knows no depth. I keep searching for you but can't find you.
You are not here but it is unimaginable that you are no longer
living. Inconceivable, unacceptable, unbelievable, surreal.

Your Mum and I are like two empty ships in the night,
passing each other but can't bear to touch each other for fear of
increasing the pain.

I miss you so much it hurts, every minute of every day.

Now Monday 7 May 2018. No better.

The end for you was not pretty but it is over now. The pain,
the confusion, the endless stream of doctors' appointments,
blood tests and pills. No more.

This picture was taken six days before you were no longer with us. You never left this bed, stood up or spoke coherently again.

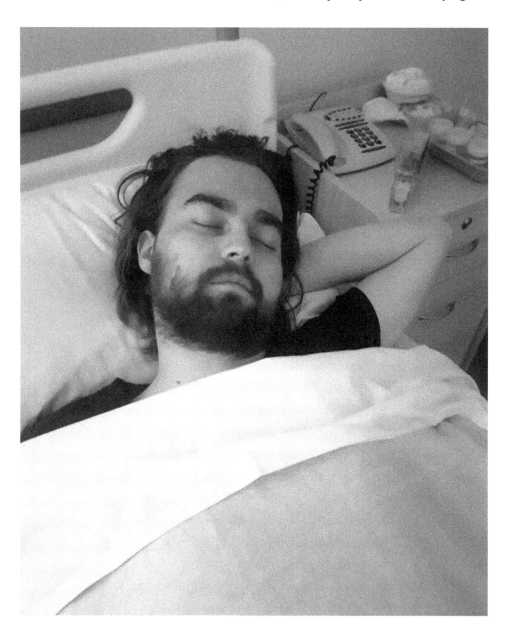

On 13 April at 5.04 pm, two days before you went, I talked to you and recorded these words:

Wish I had a pathway for getting us out of this, but I don't have any answers Jack. I don't pretend to know anything anymore. Lost any sense of direction. Probably have known for 6 weeks we've lost any sense of hope. We knew as your health deteriorated pretty obviously in front of us that nothing was working, and it was only a matter of time. Probably knew that some time ago and from day one but we pretended that we found pathways. We went on different journeys, we chased down certain rabbit holes and we had hope. We just believed at times ... we had so much passion and the smile was back on my face and I'd laugh, and I would just say that we had a chance! But we didn't.

This thing just has a life; an evil life that is beyond anything I have ever understood, comprehended or dealt with and I don't know what to do other than to sit here and talk to you and say I wish something would change, some dynamic inside you would somehow switch on and tomorrow morning find you dancing around and saying, "Dad, come on, go, we've gotta get home, gotta train for a football game!" But they are just pipe dreams, fairy dreams and that is something I'm actually very good at it because I have such a, such a rich imagination. I can pretend as much as I like but the reality is what I fear because the reality Jack is a world in which you won't belong other than as a memory and that really fucking sucks.

It's funny, you know you were quite hot a minute ago and literally, as I turned this recorder on, 2 minutes later you have actually cooled down a bit. Maybe you are listening to me; maybe something's going through but you are warmer than you should be, um, and that is infection. It is all part of the dying process so let's not pretend that we are doing anything else in the Palliative Care Ward of Saint John's Hospital. We are only here for one reason and that is make your death easy because nobody in this universe I've met so far (and I mean that I have met as I am sure people exist out there), has been able to change this dynamic. No one has been able to reverse this, and they have all just tuttered, shook their head and with a lot of knowledge and a lot of experience, said that death is inevitable, it is imminent; no one beats this disease.

Well I gave it my best shot and I just want you to know that I gave it my best shot and I would do anything, I would do anything I possibly could to reverse this, but I can't; maybe you can?

The day after you died, I was lying in bed and the first verse of a poem to you came to me. I have since finished it:

I WILL WAIT FOR YOU (JACK)

I will wait for you
Where the river meets the sea
Down past the mountains
That is where I will be

I will wait for you
No matter how long it takes
Down past the mountains
And the deep valley lakes

I will wait for you
Forever and a day
Down past the mountains
That is where I will stay

I will wait for you
I have no time
Down past the mountains
And the rows of wild thyme

I will wait for you
I have nowhere else to go
Down past the mountains
And the fields of snow

I will wait for you
Let you find your way
Down past the mountains
And cornfields of hay

I will wait for you
Alone and free
Down past the mountains
Where the river meets the sea.

Goodbye.

ASHES AND DEATH CERTIFICATE

Says it all my son. Full stop:

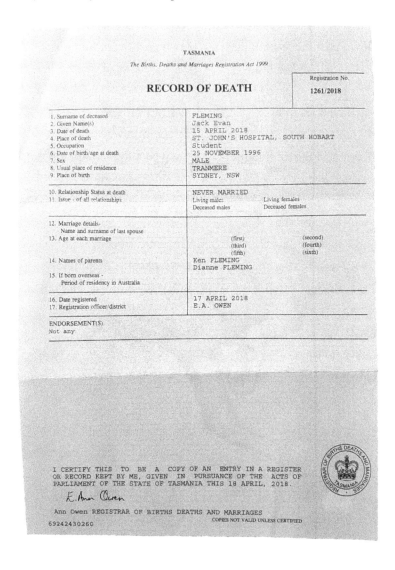

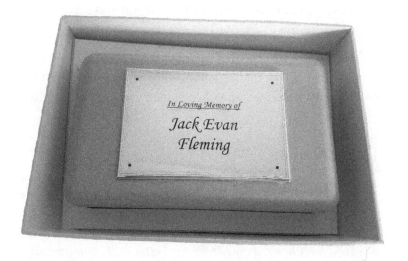

I brought your ashes home on Friday 27 April. I carried them inside and put them in your room and said to you, "You are home now son." I cried, and I cried. When Mum came home I showed her the ashes in your room.

But you are home now, where you were always comfortable and with the family that you loved.

LETTERS FROM JACK

A couple of days after your death Victoria gave us the letters you had written to us in December when it was clear to you from your writing that you knew it was over. Such beautiful words and they will haunt me forever because you are not here for me to say thank you my son, thank you. Your letter to your brothers and Mum were equally poignant and equally beautiful. Your letter to me was (unedited):

Ken

First things first, I just want you to know that the diet and everything we did/attempted okayed a major role in living as long as I did. Whatever the result, just know that what you and mum did has changed my life for the better and I can honestly say that I wouldn't have lived as along as I did (hopefully you never get this though) if it weren't for you and mum. SO THANKYOU YOU LEGENDS. Both you and mum are allowed to read this of course, it sucks that I'm having to actually write this in the first place but I trust and love both you and mum (and my family) equally.

I used to love the holiday trips we had to Binnalong Bay, Bicheno, Coles Bay, Stanley and more! The two weeks we spent in Japan were particular highlights of my life and loved every second of them! Especially the first week (with Adrian too) where I learned to snowboard! Albeit, wasn't so much fun when Chris (the rookie) crashed into me and split my leg open! The second week was great too! The third week we spent in Hong Kong was a nice experience too. Well, mainly eating all those custard breads!

I do want to also give a big thank you to your help with my university attempts at going back. You've raised an incredibly bright family and I lost my ability to read as I write this but, but I can touch type and still write quite immaculately despite not being able to read! I give kudos to your brilliance for that.

I do want to apologise for not beating this cancer, but I have no regrets in fighting this as hard as I could with you. Thanks a lot for your help, along with my family (and also my legendary friends). Just goes to show how great a father/ person you are by the impact/person you turned me into. I didn't consider giving up this fight once, and you deserve credit for that. Yourself and my amazing family and friends. Was the easiest thing I've every done turning changing my diet and working hard to live for the rest of my life with this family. Holy S**t I love this family so much and would do anything for everyone. That's how great a father you have been! I just want you to know that I could write a short thank you to everyone but I son't want to because there are so many positive things I could say about each one of my family members.

As you know there are so many great memories and things I could write, thank you so much for everything.

With love, Jack Fleming.

MUM AND I

It pains me to say things aren't good, for either of us and not good together. We can't make the other feel any better as we can't make ourselves feel any better. We are empty and have nothing but pain to give each other. But, although this will challenge us, it won't break us.

For you, for us and for everyone, we will somehow get through, but Jack it would be so much easier if you were here. But you are not, and I cannot find you.

SPERM BANK

And the final conundrum for two grieving parents, what to do
with the last remaining and alive piece of you, your sperm, that
you deposited at the beginning of this terrible journey on the
faint (and now discredited) theory that you would survive this
journey?

It came from you and it is alive, the beginning of the
dynasty you never had. We thought about donating it, to be
used by someone who unfortunately was infertile, but who
would want to take the risk of brain cancer?

But if there was a way that risk could be discounted or
removed, then someone might just have a child like you, so
happy, confident, smart and self-contained. The full package. I
don't see how that will happen but I can't bring my mind around
to destroying the last piece of this beautiful person who died so
needlessly. I can't.

And the irony is, of all my children, you were the only
one that ever talked about having children.

dedications and acknowledgements

THIS BOOK IS DEDICATED TO JACK, MY SON, AND Senator John McCain who shared the same fate and reached out to us, and to many others that have died or are suffering from glioblastoma multiforme.

I want to thank those that made this book possible and who believed that this story must be told, and to everyone that stood by Jack and this family before his death and afterwards.

I also want to particularly thank those clinicians that were involved in treating Jack and making every effort to reverse the irreversible. Particularly:

- His neurosurgeon Andrew Hunn who gave Jack time and comfort and whose brutal honesty was confronting but refreshing;

- Rosie Harrup and John Heath, his two oncologists, who exhausted every option available to deal with this disease and who tolerated my many interventions, dumb questions and layman attempts to control the treatment direction, as well as for their unabashed compassion when my eyes burned and the tears flowed;

- Victoria Jayde who felt the pain of Jack's death as strongly as his family and who guided him to write those wonderful letters before he died (and received after his death) that we will always cherish;

- The paramedics who attended our many emergencies and treated him with dignity, compassion and first-class professional care;

- The staff at the Gibson Unit (St John's Hospital) who rarely saw someone so young and who cared for him in his last week and who openly shared our family's pain and grief;

- The staff at Calvary who cared for Jack after his two major surgeries; and

- Manuel Graeber and Michael Buckland who took an interest in a stranger and gave me hope when I had none.

Finally, I want to thank Lola, our family dog, who gave Jack so much pleasure with her unquestioning love and loyalty. I think she always reserved her most vigorous tail wag for Jack, as she saw in him a kindred spirit and their bond was only broken by her death on 8 January 2018, four months before Jack succumbed to his illness. It was the first time I saw Jack cry as an adult. But sadly, it wasn't the last.

Senator John McCain

I WROTE TO SENATOR McCAIN ON 24 MAY 2018 AND got a response dated 5 June 2018. I had sent him a copy of an early draft of this manuscript (*Jack's story*) and his response was poignant, personal and compassionate. He was diagnosed with the same cancer (GBM) in July 2017 and I knew his time was short.

I was humbled by his response and Dianne and I cried when we read it. It is a beautiful message at a time of absolute tragedy in our lives and written by a father and a statesman that had come to terms with his own mortality and imminent death. It was about us and I know from reading his letter that the manuscript had affected him very deeply.

Jack, you touched his heart

JOHN McCAIN
UNITED STATES SENATOR
WASHINGTON, DC 20510

June 5, 2018

Ken Fleming

Tranmere, Tasmania

Australia 7018

Dear Mr.Fleming,

We greatly appreciate you sending the manuscript of your book. I would like to give my condolences to your family as no family should have to go through what your family endured. Taking the pain from your son's story and turning it into a moving and beautifully honest book takes a lot of courage. I appreciate the bravery it took to write this book about what it is really like inside a life with a glioblastoma multiforme. I hope this can be used to show the public how difficult cancer truly is for a person and their family. I especially appreciation the poem "I will Wait For You (Jack)." The poem was confiding and brilliant.

Again, please accept my appreciation for your generosity and your kind words, and I wish you and your family the best.

Sincerely,

John McCain

United States Senator

NOT PRINTED AT GOVERNMENT EXPENSE

Adam Lallana

A COUPLE OF DAYS AFTER JACK LEFT US I WAS rummaging through his computer and came across a partially written email to Adam Lallana, an English footballer who plays for Liverpool, my club. The letter had a number of errors but given the increasing mental challenges Jack was dealing with as the disease took its awful toll, I was surprised that he got even this far.

He died before the email was sent:

unsent email
JF ▸ ADAM LALLANA

Greetings,

My father has been helping me tremendously since I got diagnosed with brain since and I can honestly say that the only reason I have survived over 12 months is because of him. I have a frame at home but would love to get one of him signed or written anything. I don't want to be a bother. I think he would really appreciate it, just as much as I appreciate what he has done for me to fight and live this disease. To have been given only 4-5 months at most to live and to have survived 14 months so far I consider a miracle.

I watch the games all the time with him because he loves the team so much and made me a passionate number 2 supporter! Despite being a number 1 Arsenal fan haha. I already have a frame and stuff at home ready that would go with the frame. Is there, of course I will pay. I'm not sure how much longer I have to live but I can honestly say I would not have lived as long as I have without him. I even went back to uni temporarily during my diagnosis because I wanted to fight this. But Dad helped out a lot! But unfortunately it just got too hard (my brain processing) with the 2nd recurrence for me to continue. I don't know how much longer I have to live, but I wouldn't have lived as long as I have without him.

We have a signboard at home.

He was of course a Steven Gerrard favourite fan (and still is)!

(Adam Lallana T-shirt when I got diagnosed with Cancer. Signed?)

Jack Fleming and my 5 brothers and mum! We have been keeping this a secret.

I am a Liverpool tragic and a passionate supporter of Liverpool Football Club (in the UK). Adam Lallana was my idol and, until the 2017 season, I regarded him as one of the best technical players in the English Premier League. That season however he was injured and got very little game time. He was also ruled out of the England side for the 2018 World Cup due to injuries but prior to that was regarded as one of the top England footballers. I was a big fan and Jack knew that when he was well but I was

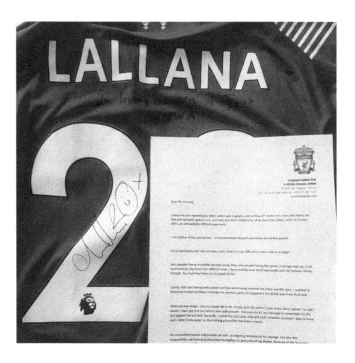

surprised that he retained that memory at the very late stages of his disease when this email was written.

I wrote to Adam and attached a copy of Jack's unfinished email to him and explained that Jack had died before he sent it and I, as his father, was finishing what Jack was unable to do. I said I would let him respond in any way he saw fit, although I didn't expect a response.

Adam wrote back (his letter was undated) and I received his response in July this year and in the parcel was a shirt that he had signed. I cried when I read his letter, as the emotions he expressed were very personal and touching.

It was a powerful message Jack, and he felt your loss almost as much as I did.

You touched his heart.

Liverpool Football Club
& Athletic Grounds Limited
PO BOX 204, Liverpool, L69 3JF
Tel: +44 (0)151 264 2500 Fax: +44 (0)151 907 9476
www.liverpoolfc.com

Dear Mr. Fleming,

I have only just received your letter, which was originally sent on May 6th earlier this year and clearly my love and sympathy goes to you, your wife and other children for what must have been, and I'm certain still is, an unimaginably difficult experience.

I am a father of two young boys – so my immediate thoughts are those of a fellow parent.

I'm so touched by the note you have sent it that it is very difficult to know where to begin.

Jack sounded like an incredibly spirited young man, who despite facing this great challenge kept joy in his heart even during those most difficult times. I have read his note back repeatedly and the humour shines through. You must have been so, so proud of him.

Clearly, with Jack having sadly passed and this note having reached me a few months later, I wanted to think how I could somehow celebrate his memory, given he supported me all the way from Australia.

There are two things I can and would like to do. Firstly, with this letter is one of my shirts signed. I'm sad I couldn't have got it to you before Jack sadly passed – but even so it's my message to remember his life and support for our club. Secondly, I would like you, your wife and Jack's brothers to know I plan to keep Jack's letter in my locker at the training ground for the entire season.

His inspirational words will provide me with an ongoing reminder of his courage, but also the responsibility we have as professional footballers to give everything always, because of the love and support of people like your Jack.

With love and compassion, You'll Never Walk Alone

Adam Lallana

Standard Chartered   new balance   BETVICTOR   Liverpool Football Club Registered Office: Anfield Road, Liverpool, L4 0TH. Company Registration Number

looking for you

ON TUESDAY 14 AUGUST 2018 I WAS IN MANLY attending an Investment Committee meeting. As usual, when I am in Sydney I have a wet lunch with my fellow Committee members. We ate at Garfish, just across from the water, and I sat at the end, next to the window.

I had a strong urge to see you. It was so powerful. I felt tears building – I had to see you again. And there, across the road you stood, looking at your phone. I called out to you in my head and you looked up and smiled, but it was not an easy smile – as if you were distracted and just being polite. You then said, "I have to go" and turned away from me and started to walk up the street. I called out to you, "Don't go, please stay with me" and you turned around and started to walk back towards me, but on the opposite side of the road. You got to the pedestrian traffic lights, waited for the lights to turn green and then crossed the road. Below me was a flowerbed and you sat on the ledge, occasionally looking up at me, smiling and then returning to your phone.

When I looked some time later you were gone. I got on a ferry back to Circular Quay, alone.

snapshots

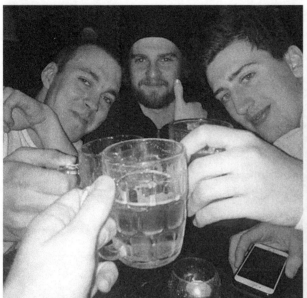 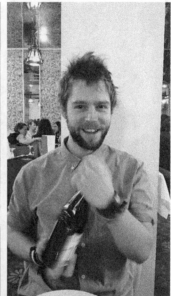

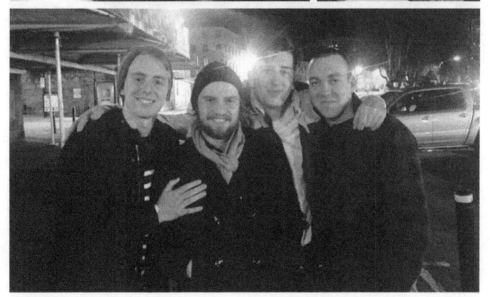

top left and above With friends, 2017   *top right Adrian 2015/16, Melbourne*

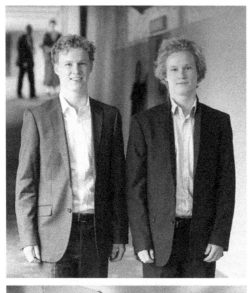
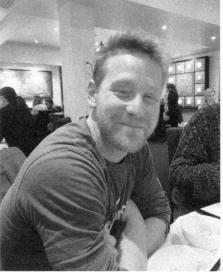
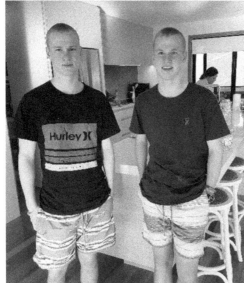
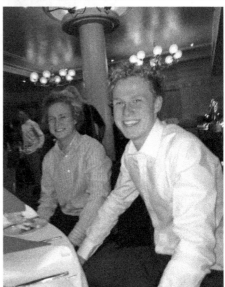

top Chris and Hugh, 2016

above Hugh and Chris shaving for brain cancer

top Stefan at Me Wah, 2016

above Hugh and Chris

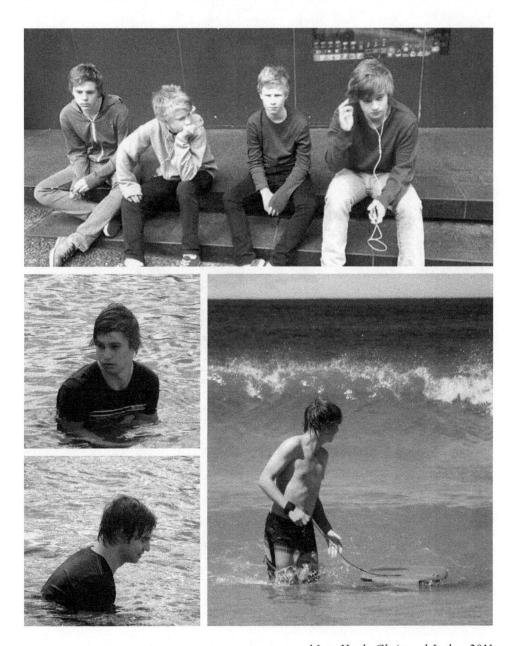

top Matt, Hugh, Chris and Jack, c 2011

above left Jack in the water! Rare moment, 2012

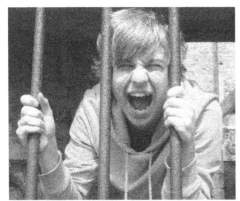
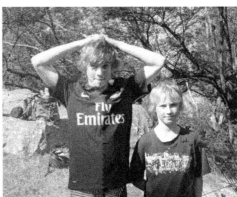
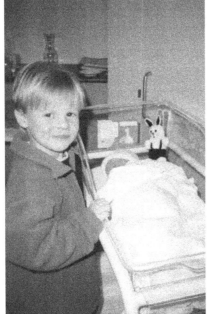
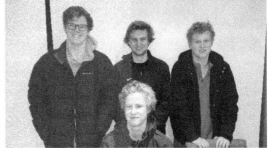
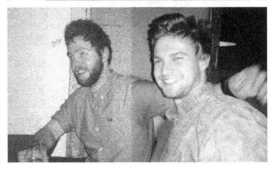

top Jack at Port Arthur

above Jack with baby Matt

top Jack and Hugh at Knocklofty

middle Matt, jack and Chris with Hugh, sitting

above Adrian and Jack, Melbourne, 2015

(before it all turned to shit)

CPSIA information can be obtained
at www.ICGtesting.com
Printed in the USA
BVHW011621030222
627785BV00016B/308

9 780648 703211